"Into the often terrifying worl[d of type 1 diabetes come these] remarkable dogs and the equa[lly remarkable people who] train them. Meet them all in this book, which is not only a wonderful resource for people living with diabetes but a source of sensitivity training for the rest of us. You will cry along with the families but also rejoice with them as they discover the seemingly miraculous Wildrose Way."

—Donna Levine, Copy Chief, *Garden & Gun* magazine

"These dogs' sense of smell and their ability to work is just amazing."
—Grayson Schaffer, Senior Editor, *Outside* magazine

"I had never realized what a devastating illness type 1 diabetes can be and had never heard of Diabetic Alert Dogs (DADs) until reading *Lifesaving Labradors*. These personal narratives by owners of DADs, collected and edited by Ben McClelland, are both informative and deeply moving, and should be widely read by those in the medical profession, by sufferers from diabetes and their families, and by anyone who seeks knowledge and understanding. All praises to the lifesaving dogs and to the wonderful breeders and trainers at Mississippi's Wildrose Kennels."

—Ann Fisher-Wirth, co-editor, *The Ecopoetry Anthology*

"Ben McClelland's book is masterfully thorough as an all-around primer about service dogs in general. Readers experience just the right amount of amazement balancing the pure facts of what canine attendants can do for humans with tricky physical conditions. This book bridges the divide between science and compassion, and the reader comes out knowing what to do and why. Interested in service dogs? Read this book first."

—Diane Carey, author of *How to Help Stray Pets and Not Get Stuck*

Lifesaving Labradors:
Stories From Families With Wildrose Diabetic Alert Dogs

Edited by Ben McClelland

© Copyright 2014 by Ben McClelland

ISBN 978-1-938467-90-5

All rights reserved. No part of this publication may be reproduced, stored in a retrieval system, or transmitted in any form or by any means – electronic, mechanical, photocopy, recording, or any other – except for brief quotations in printed reviews, without the prior written permission of the author.

Published by

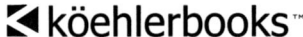 köhlerbooks™

210 60th Street
Virginia Beach, VA 23451
212-574-7939

On the cover: Charlie and Lily Simonton.
Photo by Deanna Whitehead.

www.lifesavinglabradors.com

A portion of the proceeds from this book will be used to support diabetes organizations

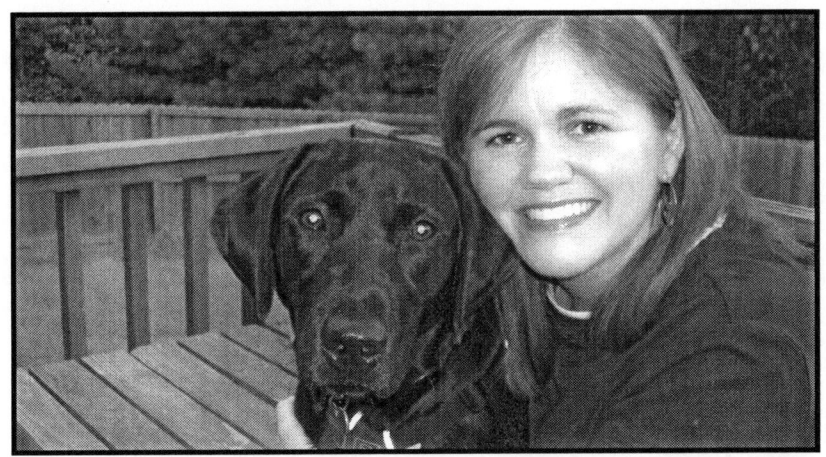

LIFESAVING LABRADORS

Stories From Families With Wildrose Diabetic Alert Dogs

Edited by
Ben McClelland

VIRGINIA BEACH
CAPE CHARLES

Table of Contents

Mike Stewart: *Foreword*	2
Ben McClelland: *Masters of Scent*	5
Rachel Thornton: *A Mother's Quest*	13
Mr Darcy and Abi Thornton Atkinson: *At Work Daily*	23
Teddy Bear and Capri and Ciara Smith: *Communal Knowledge*	41
Olive and Devon Wright: *Team Empathy*	75
Juniper and Megan DeHaven: *Special Communication*	91
Gracie and Sharon Stinson: *Miracles and Misunderstandings*	109
Charlie, Lily and Angie Simonton: *Focus in School Settings*	119
Keeper and Kitty and Anna Grace Berry: *Our Journey*	133
Hatch and Duane V. Miller: *Multitasking*	145
Willow Wonka and Adam and Laurie Schwartz: *Redundant Systems*	159
Drake and Tom Arsenault with Lisa Mayer: *Urban Dog Hero*	181
Training Tips for DADs	192
When Does Training Begin?	211
Notes on Contributors	256

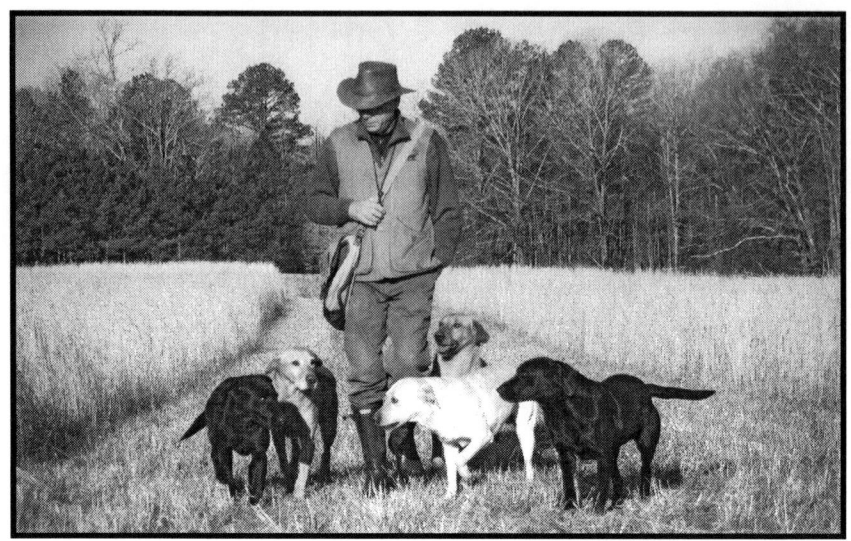

Foreword

Historically, man has benefitted from the companionship of the first domesticated animal, the dog. Dogs first teamed with humans as scavengers and hunters, ultimately to evolve into separate breeds and crosses with diverse capabilities. "Man's best friend" so accurately describes these beloved canine companions with the amazing ability to serve a range of roles, relying on compatibility, intelligence, instinct, and of course, a keen sense of smell. I am confident that the field of canine training and behavioral study has only just begun to tap the vast competencies of dogs.

One such exemplar is the Diabetic Alert Dog (DAD). We refer to the Wildrose DAD as the *Master of Scent*. Training a Wildrose British Labrador as an alert dog certainly qualifies as amazing—even a bit mysterious. These animals actually predict a swing in a diabetic's blood sugar well before other indicators. An obvious indicator is scenting—*The nose knows!* But are there other, subtler body changes the perceptive dog may identify? Therein lies the mystery.

At Wildrose, we specialize in the British Labradors highly valued for their temperament, moderate size, retrieving and natural game-finding abilities. These fine dogs has been selectively bred for more than 150 years as game-finders, so their scenting abilities are quite keen and highly refined, perfect scent discriminators. Thanks to outstanding genetics and the hard work of the many DAD trainers and volunteers, who intensively train the dogs for service work, these exceptional Labradors are changing the lives of people with Type 1. Moreover, as the stories in this collection demonstrate, DAD team families are dedicated to working with canine service companions to help manage the health care of their diabetics.

I have enjoyed a lifetime of training dogs for companionship, game location and recovery, as well as outside adventurers, but the DAD training experience has been a most rewarding, yet challenging, journey. It is one thing to train a dog to bring back a game bird that would have otherwise been lost. It's quite another to participate in developing a canine that possesses the ability to save a life—or at the very least, to help a person become more independent and enjoy the confidence to lead a normal life. That is the mission of the Wildrose DAD.

Join the journey as you explore the challenges, mysteries, and wonders that unfold in these dramatic stories of Labrador service dogs—trained the *Wildrose Way*—and their diabetic partners whose lives these unbelievable animals have blessed.

Mike Stewart
Wildrose Kennels

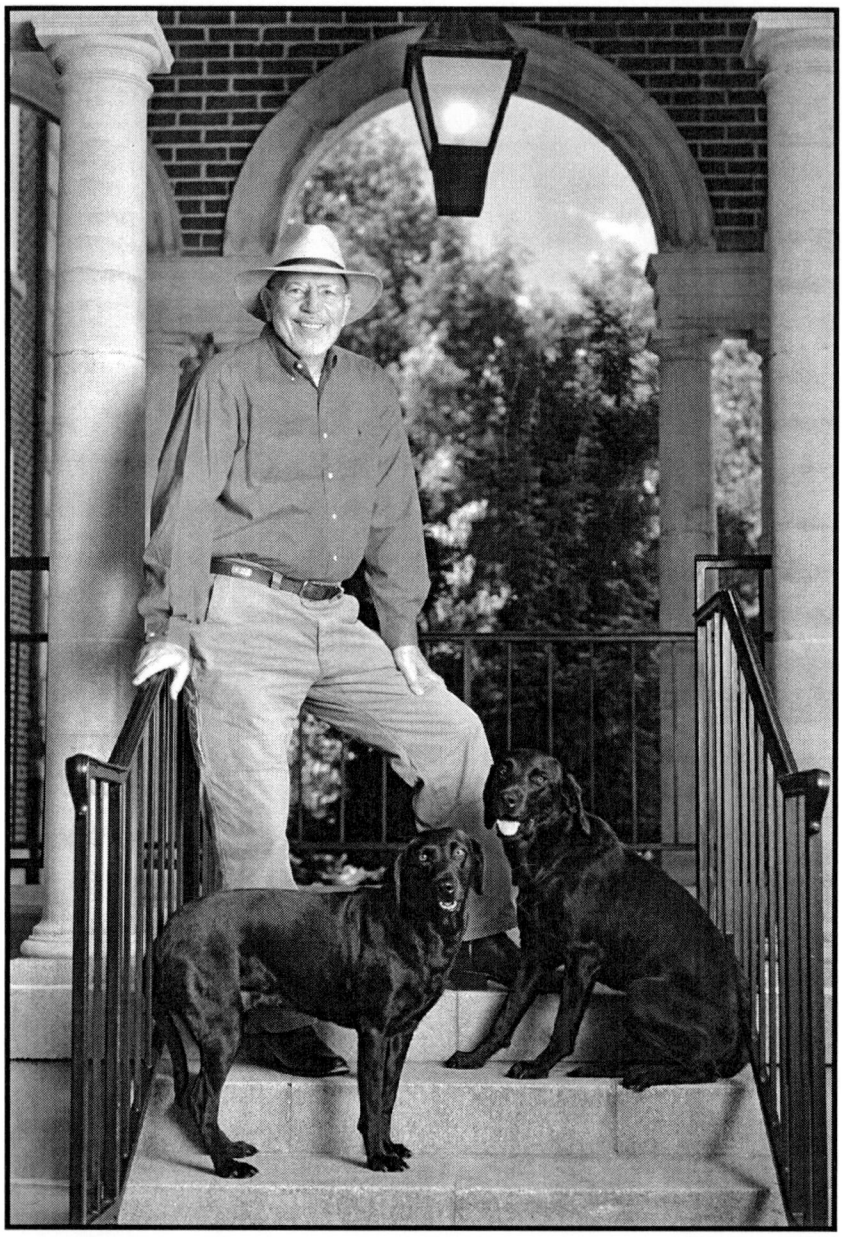

Ben McClelland shown with Eider and Mac on the steps of Bondurant Hall, The University of Mississippi.

Ben McClelland:
Masters of Scent

IT'S JUST A DOG KENNEL, like some you've no doubt visited. But it's so much more. They're just ordinary folks here, like you and me. Yet there's something very different about them.

This is Mike and Cathy Stewart's Wildrose, a haven for British Labradors, tucked away in the piney hills of northern Mississippi, Faulkner's renowned landscape. Hundreds of people visit here annually to pick up pups from the celebrated genetic lines. Most are gundog enthusiasts or outdoor adventure seekers who want steady, well-trained companions at home and afield. But petite Texan Angie Simonton also visited with Lily, her blonde preschooler. College sophomore Devon Wright, a competitive equestrian, and her mother flew in from Colorado for a look. Capri Smith, a savvy romance novelist, brought daughter Ciara on an overland journey for some training with their dog, Teddy Bear. Megan DeHaven took time away from her demanding job to drive down from Ohio. Twentysomething Sharon Stinson and husband Jeremy came for Gracie. And several others like them have also visited in the last few years. Yes, these people would fit in with us at, say, a summer picnic or at a family reunion or at an afternoon concert in the park. But something significant sets them apart. Little Lily, athletic Devon, sweet Ciara, pixie-haired Megan, and tall, demure Sharon are all type 1 diabetics, an affliction that used to be known as juvenile diabetes. Like three million other Americans they suffer from an autoimmune disease that destroys the beta cells in the pancreas responsible for producing insulin. Death cast its shadow over each of them.

They all came to Wildrose seeking diabetic alert dogs to hold death at bay. To get here they traveled a path that pioneer Rachel Thornton had cleared for them. Rachel and her very ill eleven-year-old daughter, Abi, toughed it out, training Mr Darcy to alert for Abi. Then Rachel and Wildrose owners, Mike and Cathy Stewart, created opportunities for other diabetics and their caregivers to use dogs as medical assistants to help them monitor their levels of blood sugar (also referred to as blood glucose or BG) and live more normal lives.

Because these folks look healthy, it's hard for us to understand the medical challenges that they face every day. Imagine that, willy-nilly, your blood sugar level could rise or fall suddenly because your pancreas no longer works to supply insulin. What's worse, you can neither predict these changes, nor can you feel any side effects—until you are dangerously sick. With a high level you might experience febrile convulsions. With a low one, you would likely fall unconscious.

Consider the effect that this condition would have on your daily life. You could suffer an attack while swimming, riding a bike, or driving a car. You could be enjoying dinner and a movie with friends. Or you could be sound asleep in the middle of the night. Because these incidents could occur at any time and might have severe consequences, you might choose to reduce your activities and try to stay safe at home. You might become reclusive or depressed. Diabetics suffer from lack of insulin production, which can lead to sudden changes in blood sugar levels. Many things contribute to sugar levels, from emotions to exercise, from eating carbohydrates to getting a cold. Several times emergency responders rushed Sharon Stinson to the hospital when she fell into diabetic comas. All of the parents in this group, around-the-clock caregivers for their children, have frantically administered Glucagon shots or force-fed sugar drinks in desperate attempts to steady erratic glycemic events. Like Capri Smith, all of them have gone on daredevil car rides to the ER, desperate to save their daughters' lives. "Battling diabetes is an unimaginable fight. Every day," Kitty Berry attests "The fight requires every bit of energy and faith we can muster."

Monitoring blood sugar levels is an unrelenting task for type 1 diabetics and their caregivers. The goal is to maintain tight control over the glycemic range, minimizing fluctuations so as to maintain normal activities and to prevent any of the several harmful side effects of wide, erratic sugar swings. Even with modern insulin monitoring and delivery systems, type 1 diabetics continue to struggle to achieve healthy monthly averages, a key to long-term health.

A diabetic alert dog, known as a DAD, is a tool in diabetes management. Each dog is trained to notify the diabetic or the caregiver of low and high blood sugar levels, thereby allowing them to promptly make necessary corrections to avert the episode or lessen its severity. A hypo- or hyperglycemic attack can lead to a seizure, coma, or death, making these well-trained dogs true lifesavers. The DAD's performance can result in tighter glycemic control, which decreases the likelihood of devastating, long-term complications, including kidney failure, retinopathy, neuropathy, and heart disease.

As these diabetics and their caregivers struggled with this relentless disease, they turned to dogs as effective monitors of blood sugar changes. Mr Darcy, Teddy Bear, Olive, Gracie, Ruby, Charlie, Keeper, Willow, Juniper, Drake, and Hatch—these canines are the masters of scent, the heroes of their owners' real-life dramas. These DADs consistently alert their owners to sugar level changes more frequently and sooner than the mechanical monitors that the diabetics wear. Some report that dog alerts are twenty minutes ahead of the monitors; some, as much as an hour ahead. What do these precious minutes mean to the diabetic or her caregiver? In the case of rapidly falling blood levels, it can enable one to take preventive action to head off a precipitous drop before it plunges dangerously low.

How does the dog monitor changes in blood sugar level? When some people first hear about diabetic alert dogs, they are in awe at the dogs' ability to "smell." Others are skeptical. Dr. Dana Hardin, of Eli Lilly and Company, is conducting research into the special scenting abilities of DADs to discover scientific evidence of the volatile organic compounds that dogs smell emanating from a diabetic's body in, for example, perspiration, breath, and saliva. We have long known that dogs possess a superior olfactory system. Relying on their keen scenting capabilities, trainers have employed dogs to seek out cached drugs, lost hikers, shed antlers, and arson accelerants. As hunting dogs are trained to follow the scent of wild game and drug-detection dogs are trained to sniff out concealed illegal drugs, DADs are trained to smell changes in human scent when a diabetic's blood sugar level changes. Current research on canine olfaction reveals a complex, sophisticated method of knowing the world by smell. Dogs know us primarily by smell, using extensive nasal passages and odor-collection chambers, as well as the nasal vomeronasal organ, a special sac "covered with more receptor sites for molecules." Dogs recognize us by our unique odors—by our sweat, perfume, and clothing. They can tell if we've just bathed and what food or drink we've recently had. And as our storywriters reveal, DADs smell, sense, know their team members' sugar levels.

Still, dogs' ability to know us goes beyond this phenomenal sense of smell. Dogs are vigilant, keenly observing their human companions' behavior. They read us. Not only can they understand our mood from our body language and facial expression, but they also perceive our emotions, smell our fear, sense our enthusiasm, and feel our sadness. Devon Wright explains the occasional need for restorative action when she and Olive feed too intensely on each other's emotions: "I had no idea how much Olive fed off my energy until I met Rachel at the airport that year. I was obviously emotional when Olive was leaving, but I sat down with Rachel and talked for a while. Rachel observed that as I calmed, Olive followed. This was a reminder of how attentive Oli is to me. It is one of her strongest qualities, but it can also be a negative if she stresses because I do." In a brief vacation away from Devon, Olive was able to gain balance in a reset period and return to work with her more aware handler, Devon.

Hundreds of people have attested to the healing power of companion dogs and their uncanny ability to detect illnesses, including cancers. Researcher Sharon Sakson recounts the stories of dogs who have helped hundreds of people, including assist dogs for the disabled, cancer detection dogs, and therapy dogs.

Notably, in the service alert dog field more and more families are living with attendant dogs. On the rise in particular are the numbers of trained DADs. Wildrose, already renowned as a premier breeding and training kennel for gundogs and adventure dogs, developed a nonprofit program to train and place DADs with diabetic clients. Now these Labradors are changing the lives of people with Type I diabetes across the United States.

Wildrose's Diabetic Alert Dog Program rests on the same positive training philosophy as the Gentleman's Gundog and Adventure Dog Programs. It gets its integrity from Mike Stewart's expertise as dog trainer; he designed the training regimen that each dog follows. Stewart's recent book, *Sporting Dog and Retriever Training The Wildrose Way*, has set the standard for gundog training, a benchmark of excellence that Stewart has already demonstrated in his numerous training workshops, videos, and DVDs. The obedience-training regimen for DADs is based on the same training philosophy and practices, known widely as the Wildrose Way. In addition, Rachel Thornton developed the scent-training program for the DADs at Wildrose. Their Labradors possess instinctive scenting ability and a biddable temperament, both of which suit them well for this service work. About her DAD, Megan DeHaven states, "Juniper's ability to alert me has given me the help that I needed to get my diabetes back into a good control… Because she is able to alert me so well, I have been consistently improving. With her alerts she has been able to wake me from sleep when I have been having dangerously low or high blood sugar. She has been able to make me aware when my blood sugar is beginning to become dangerous while I have been driving so I can pull over and treat the situation… She endures my long work hours and strange shifts, while consistently alerting for my needs. She has helped me handle the burden of managing a very complicated disease. She has saved my life."

This collection of dog stories—narratives about getting, training, and living with a dog—reveal that a dog that has an invisible, seemingly magical power. Still, these stories also reveal the unvarnished truth, the ups and downs, of daily life with an animal in the household—a domesticated animal, to be sure, but one that needs constant oversight from the team leader. As they report in their stories, Angie, Devon, Megan and the other handlers participate in daily exercises and play activities that keep their DADs mentally sharp and in focus, while having fun.

Because the stories of DADs involve families—often with very young diabetic children like Lily, Faith, and Anna Grace—in medical crises, the narratives present dramatic scenes of people experiencing intense emotion: fear, desperation, anguish, and then hope, relief, assurance, and gratitude. These emotionally charged DAD stories reveal powerful human dramas as they unfold, dense with the real stuff of everyday lives—well, everyday lives that are tasked with the considerable challenges of serious medical conditions. Lily Simonton's mother, Angie, said, "I truly believe it is hard for people outside of the family to understand the gravity of diabetes and then to understand the level of care and security these amazing dogs provide." This collection of stories presents an inside-the-family understanding of this grave disease and the life-transforming abilities of these diabetic alert dogs. Yes, dogs from Wildrose, a place that's so much more than a kennel. And ordinary folks, who are doing extraordinary things with their dogs.

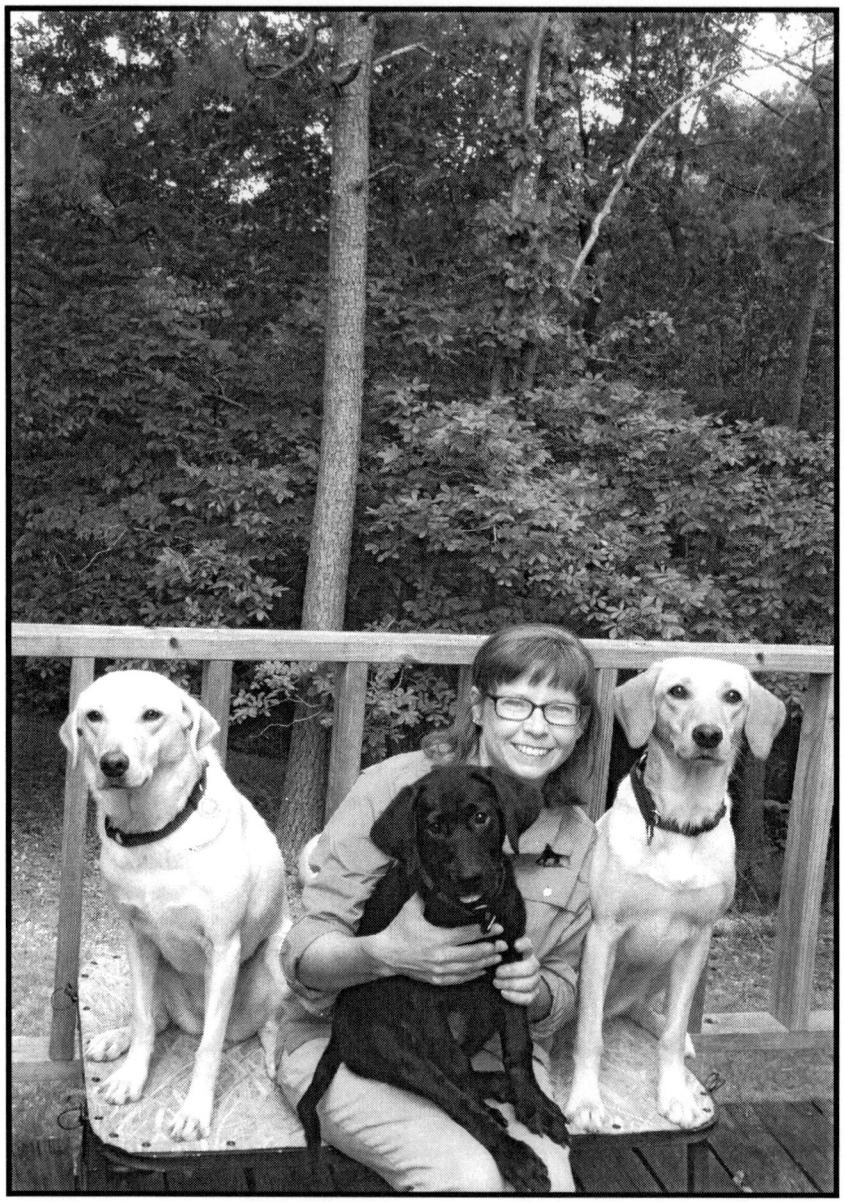

Rachel Thorton with Hope, Silas, and Ezri.

Rachel Thornton: A Mother's Quest

IN 2004 I WAS BUSILY engaged with my pastor-husband in raising our seven children, when Abi, our fourth child, became ill—very ill. It was a busy time when our family was facing many changes: My husband, Mark, had just been deployed as a chaplain to Iraq. We had moved ourselves from the parsonage where we had lived, to another home in Hamilton, Alabama. It was holidays. We stayed up late at night and we had been eating a lot of holiday food. I figured my eleven-year-old was dealing with a lot of stress. So, initially, I dismissed her sporadic sicknesses as perhaps a stomach virus. Maybe she picked it up from a friend. I overlooked some symptoms, such as a yeast infection that wouldn't go away. Had I known more at the time, I would have seen that as an indication of too much sugar in her urine.

Abi's vomiting became more frequent and much more intense. She lost twenty pounds. My little stick of a girl lost so much weight. She was thirsty all of the time, and even though hunger plagued her, she always threw up after eating. She became embarrassed to be with her friends or in public when it was mealtime. Some people cruelly joked that she might be bulimic.

Unable to get a good diagnosis of Abi's condition, we watched her decline, eventually into a coma. Only a rushed emergency room visit and the incidental observation by a doctor that they passed saved Abi's life. That night we began a long journey of finding a way to manage Abi's unpredictable disease: type 1 diabetes.

At home we tackled this project with fervor. Since we are a home-schooling family, we are used to activity-based educational endeavors. Each day we threw ourselves into managing Abi's condition. Because she is highly motivated and independent, Abi performed quite well, keeping a chart of her blood level, maintaining a good diet, staying on time with her insulin injections, and eventually managing an insulin pump, which she programmed to give a regulated delivery of insulin. Abi was not to be deterred. Around her twelfth birthday, after we got a new endocrinologist and her first pump, Abi went straight into a softball game. We felt that she had gotten a grip on this situation.

Shortly after Mark returned home, our sense of comfort was suddenly and violently shaken. One night in April when we were enjoying our church's week of revival, Abi, who always had an exceptional voice, sang for the service.

We returned home and went to bed with a sense of wellbeing. We checked Abi's blood level at midnight and again at two. We went back to sleep, planning to check it again at four.

But at three o'clock we were roused in the dark of the night by a strange noise. An unnatural commotion intruded on the sounds of the peaceful river flowing in our backyard, the chirping crickets, and the croaking frogs. They were noises I'd never heard before, noises that are indelibly imprinted into my soul: crashing and thrashing and guttural moaning coming from Abi. Rushing in, we found her locked in a seizure writhing on the floor moaning. Oh, that sound! My baby's beautiful angelic voice had become a monstrous animal noise. With her eyes rolled back in her head, Abi's entire body twitched and jerked in convulsions.

We grabbed her, shook her, and began yelling at her, trying to revive her. We knew to get sugar into her quickly, but she was fighting us. We dribbled juice along the inside of her cheek. Slowly, she began to respond, to go limp, as we stabilized her. When she came to, Abi said, "Daddy, where are you?" She was blind. For ten long minutes, she couldn't see.

How could this have happened so suddenly? As I held her after this trauma, I had no idea that we could expect this to happen at any time, especially at night. Families of diabetics talk about the dead-in-the-bed syndrome. I had read from the American Diabetes Association and the Juvenile Diabetic Research Fund that one in twenty diabetics die from low blood sugar episodes, causing a condition called hypoglycemia.

For Mark that night was his first experience with the gravity of the disease. "I didn't understand it until those fretful minutes in the early dawn," he explained. "I knew she had it and that it was serious, but until that time, it was just something I watched Abi manage. And she managed it well. She checked with her meter; she dosed herself with her pump; she changed her pump. Until that night, I was just the one that paid for and picked up the supplies. But, in those minutes, it became very personal to me."

"Grand mal seizure. Nighttime hypoglycemia," the ER doctor calmly explained.

"The post-traumatic stress I experienced from Abi's episode is greater than anything I experienced in all my years of service—two wars and recovery efforts at the World Trade Center and at Katrina. At that point, I began to fear what would happen during the night while Abi slept; I knew that she needed some mechanism to alert her—and us—to overnight hypoglycemia,"

Mark concluded.

My husband and I would scour the earth to find something to help prevent this from happening again. We would not calmly accept this as just another facet of type 1 diabetes. We would find an answer.

✳ ✳ ✳

Desperation drove us in search of anything to warn us of dangerous blood sugar fluctuations. The continuous glucose monitor, a subcutaneous sensor that gives blood sugar updates at five-minute intervals, was a new device at that time, but not approved for minors and not approved by our insurance. So it was not an option. The search seemed futile until I read something about a young lady with a dog that could sense the changes in her BG levels—a diabetic alert dog.

We soon learned that a trained dog was very costly. We raised eight thousand dollars to donate to an organization that offered training for diabetic alert dogs and their handlers. Our family, friends, and community responded generously. Unwittingly and very unfortunately, we chose the wrong organization.

It would take us several months to discover this scam and a couple more years to rectify the situation. Many of us families that felt abused and swindled were included in a lawsuit that an attorney filed against the organization. At the attorney general's proceedings against the unscrupulous businessperson, our experts testified on our behalf: our dog demonstrated no evidence of scent training, no evidence of drive to do scent work, and no temperament to be a service dog.

My daughter was devastated. The dog, Eggo, was pitifully frightened of everyone and everything. A dog who is fearful is a dangerous thing. In an effort to protect herself, Eggo displayed significant levels of aggression. Abi had earned her trust, but Abi was the only one she trusted. Eggo growled, lunged and snapped at anyone who came near her. Because Abi was determined to do everything she could to help Eggo, she began to seclude herself and Eggo in her bedroom. In this way, Eggo was happy and safe. But Abi was not safe. Eggo could not alert. She could not perform any task other than attempting to keep herself safe from the many ghosts in her head. Abi still had wildly fluctuating blood glucose levels that she was unable to detect on her own. At night—or any time that I needed to enter Abi's room for a BG check—I was greeted by a crouching, growling, frightened canine who was recoiled in a corner, with her teeth bared, ready to attack. The dog whom we had picked up to assist my daughter was actually creating much more danger than we had ever known. Yet, Abi's efforts to provide for Eggo's safety began to create something akin to a dysfunctional co-dependency. Abi knew that Eggo depended on her and no one else, and because of this, the connection between Abi and Eggo was strong, thick and deep. When we were required to return Eggo, the separation was devastating for Abi. Absolutely devastating.

In August 2010, we won a judgment against the business that was shut down. However, none of us ever recovered the money that others had invested for us. We had also lost precious time and had wasted the money that our friends, family, and community had tirelessly raised. Worst of all, Abi had no dog. The experience had wounded our confidence in service dogs' ability to perform this task. Nonetheless, we were determined to pick up the pieces. Research renewed our confidence in the dogs' ability to scent. At that time there were very few trainers of diabetic alert dogs and scarcely any that were willing to share any information with us. With no industry oversight or standards and no confirmation of skills or training methods, I feared a repeat of our past nightmare, but I was much more fearful of the unrelenting villain that was robbing my daughter of her health and confidence. I immersed myself in details about canine scent discrimination and diabetes itself. I continued to contact anyone who would take time to talk to me on either topic: the dog's nose or the physiological details of diabetic events.

One positive outcome of our experience with the fiasco was that the core group of diabetics and their families bonded and continued a social network beyond the Missouri case settlement. We decided that the road to obtaining a medical assistance dog could not dead-end there. We were committed to helping our sick children. And many of us felt obliged to forge ahead on behalf of the people who had donated to us. And so we began researching further. We placed calls all over the country and even into foreign countries. We talked to every type of canine scent discrimination expert who would answer our questions. We met with dog trainers from several states. We shared, sifted, purged, and combined information to formulate a plan of action: We would train our own diabetic alert dogs.

Through a serendipitous connection with someone from that group, we came upon a new group of pups from a Wildrose Kennels' line. Knowing that the pups came out of a trusted bloodline, we hired an experienced trainer to examine the pups for soundness, temperament, and scenting ability. Capri Smith and I were each blessed to get pups from this litter, as were some other families. Remaining members in our group also found dogs from other sources.

The next step was turning pups into diabetic alert dogs and turning us moms into dog handlers. We formed our own little think tank, brainstorming various training ideas. We organized a weeklong training session, hired the trainer who had examined the pups, and planned to develop protocols for training diabetic alert dogs. In February 2008 we convened at a home in Dallas and worked for a week on obedience and scenting scenarios.

Members of our group developed some novel training techniques. After having used a diabetic's sweaty sock or her clothes, we handlers searched for scent that would be purer, less contaminated by external factors. We began using sterile gauze pads containing saliva samples. We placed saliva samples in salt-and-pepper shaker bottles and hid them around the training room along with some empty bottles. When a dog went to a shaker and sniffed a sample bottle, his handler gave him a treat. During a session, my daughter's dog, Mr Darcy, sniffed a sample and walked directly over to Abi. I checked her and sure enough, Abi's blood sugar was low. I cried. This nine-week-old pup got it; he got it. Thus began our diabetic-alert-dog training regimen, details of which appear in the book's final section.

Mr Darcy succeeded at learning scent work because he had such strong drive. However, that same get-up-and-go made him a real challenge with some obedience tasks.

I telephoned Cathy Stewart and informed her that we had a pup from early Wildrose progeny. In several phone consultations we talked about Mr Darcy, and she invited us to visit Wildrose for a puppy picking in October 2008. After their workshop and send-off of new owners and their pups, Cathy and Mike sat down with Abi, Mr Darcy, and me. Mike worked with Abi and Mr Darcy on obedience.

Afterward, he turned to me and asked, "What else do you need me to do?"

"Help my friends," I said immediately. "There are more like me. Lots more."

So Mike and Cathy put their considerable know-how into service for many of us who had been run over in our journey to find trained dogs. That year Wildrose hosted the first open diabetic alert dog conference for handlers and dogs. Since then Wildrose has hosted several more annual conferences, each of which has grown steadily.

At the first conference, attendees were astounded at the temperament and obedient demeanor of the Wildrose-trained dogs. One family dared to ask Mike to train a "Mr Darcy" for their little girl. Not long after that Cathy called me to come pick up a small black pup. I was to start his training for this little girl.

How thrilling! A worthy diabetic-alert-dog training program was born, the Wildrose Service Companions, a legal nonprofit. Since then we have gained considerable support from individuals and groups. Because the demand for trained diabetic alert dogs far outstrips our ability to raise and train such dogs, we have developed an application system, whereby families complete extensive information forms, explaining their medical and home situation.

This program began with Mr Darcy, Abi's fox-red British Lab. Because of Mr Darcy's success, we have been able to share information and education and encouragement through www.diabeticalertdog.com. When I became the head trainer for the Wildrose program, I was catapulted into a role for which I felt woefully ill-equipped. Seeking to educate myself and enrich my experience, I became a certified clicker trainer through the Karen Pryor Academy and pursued an animal behavior course with Dr. Susan Friedman. I also sought out experts in canine scent discrimination and traveled to study and learn. And, significantly, I learned much from Mike Stewart, just as he learned much from Abi and Mr Darcy.

One afternoon on the lawn at Wildrose, when we were working with Mr Darcy, Mike Stewart coined a phrase that is now commonplace in the diabetic-alert-dog world. As Mike observed Mr Darcy's keen focus on Abi, he looked at me in his typical no-nonsense manner and said, "We have to call them something; we'll call them DADs." The term "DAD" caught on like wildfire. Thanks to Abi and Mr Darcy, Wildrose Kennels has blazed a trail in many aspects of the DAD world.

Even though DADs are an unproven and often-contested type of service dog, I wait faithfully for research to validate the work that is being done. In the meantime, I have personal validation. We have documented Mr Darcy's training and his service to Abi in alerting to low BG, high BG, and also alerting when ketones are present. His trained indication is to retrieve and hold a "bringsel" in his mouth, while offering additional discriminatory signals based upon whether her BG is low or high.

As a result of Mr Darcy's vigilant companionship, Abi has not had any seizures when he was with her. On two occasions when she was rushed to the hospital for emergency procedures— and separate from Mr Darcy— she experienced seizures at the hospital. This is powerful validation of his indispensible on-going service for Abi. Her A1C, a blood test that gives an indication of the average blood sugar level over a four-month-period, has improved. Her glycemic range has improved, with fewer lows, fewer highs, and staying closer to her target value. Mr Darcy gives Abi advance warning on most occasions so that many lows are completely eliminated and so that most highs are addressed before they are extreme.

We have charted and graphed his alerts; he indeed provides a more proactive rather than reactive approach to diabetic management. On many occasions his nose reacts to the odor prior to the meter detecting data from the blood.

Mr Darcy has increased Abi's confidence. Even though Abi is unable to remember actual seizures, she can recall and is greatly shaken by the feeling of the onset of a seizure and the feeling of total helplessness before and after them. And she has heard stories about what happens during them. The imminent threat and the unpredictability, even when diligently doing all the right things, caused her to lose confidence and become less social for fear of "what if." No teenager wants to seize when they are out with a group of friends. Furthermore, Abi developed a fear of going to sleep, because that was a time when she would be completely vulnerable and totally out of control.

Mr Darcy alerts at home, in public, when she is driving, and when she is sleeping. Mr Darcy sleeps right beside Abi in bed, 'watching' over her blood sugar levels vigilantly all through the night. He is her constant and faithful companion. As a service dog, he is permitted to go anywhere she goes. She has gracefully navigated many milestones with Mr Darcy: completing high school, recording music in a Nashville studio, participating in church choir each Sunday, leading in worship, driving, courting, taking outings with friends, attending college, living in an off-campus apartment with a friend, working in Financial Aid office on campus, getting married, and giving birth to her daughter. Mr Darcy's alerting is stellar in any situation because Abi trained with those goals in mind and his training was constant and consistent in a wide array of venues.

In a figurative sense and in a real sense as well, he alone is able to bear the burden of this disease as intimately as she.

No, the laboratory documented scientific proof is not available concerning diabetic alert dogs, but I have empirical data. I have a healthy child. Abi has a changed life. Mr Darcy is an invaluable tool. He takes care of his girl—our girl—who had been so terribly ill, keeping her glycemic range in bounds, improving her quality of life, and extending her length of life, too. He's also the reason that Wildrose Service Companions came into existence, providing so many others with a DAD.

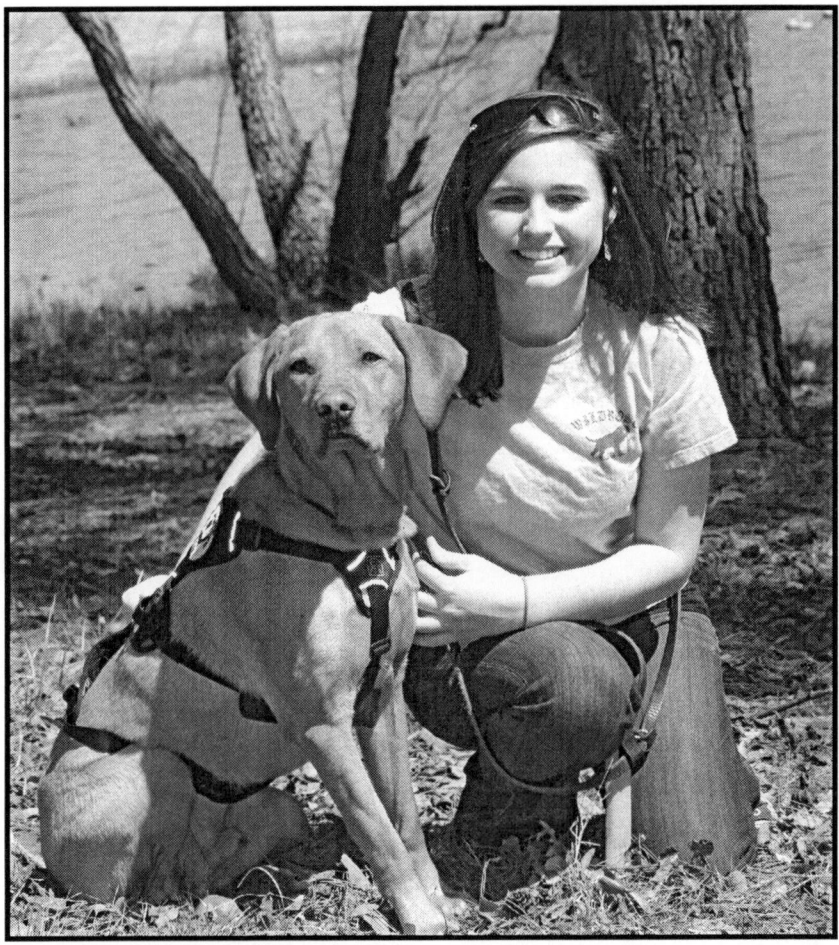

Mr Darcy with Abi Atkinson.

Mr Darcy and Abi Thornton Atkinson: At Work Daily

IN 2004 WE MOVED INTO a new home in Hamilton, Alabama, where I spent my days with my younger sisters. The Buttahatchee River ran through the woods in back of our house and my mom loved to sit on a big rock while my sisters and I rode floats down the rapids and tried to catch fish with disposable cups. Occasionally there would be a snake sighting, and I would retreat into the house for several weeks until I had forgotten about it. Around Christmas when I was eleven years old, I started getting sick. My symptoms included sleeping an abnormal length of time. Then I began to get sick after each meal. My flu-like illness progressed until I was finally diagnosed with type 1 diabetes. In trying to cope with my disease, my mother searched the Internet and learned about dogs that could alert diabetics to blood sugar drops.

One winter day we drove to the dog training business that we eventually found to be an enormous scam. I was given a dog that had been found at an animal shelter only a few months earlier. She had no training whatsoever. She wasn't even housebroken. After returning home we struggled with her for too long, because she started lunging, growling, and barking at strangers in public and at home. We finally returned her.

The ordeal destroyed me emotionally. Despite this dog's bad temperament and lack of training, I had bonded with her. Because of her aggressive behavior, I had to keep her in my room with me at all times. I spent hours with her, talking to her, holding her, taking her for walks, telling her my secrets and my feelings. I worked with her so hard, fully believing that one day she would get over all of her problems and I could train her to alert me to my blood sugar levels. I had perfect faith that she loved me enough to work out her problems. But I was wrong. The dog had to go. She became a danger to my family. She would lunge for my little brother and try to bite my dad. She loved me, but hated everyone else. This dog that I had sacrificed my time and money for, the dog I fell head over heels in love with, was a disaster.

I was angry. But more than anything, I was sad. I thought I had found a cure for my seizures. I thought I had found something that would let me sleep at night. After all the work, months, and money I still had the same questions and the same problems.

After all I had been through, I hadn't found any answers.

My mom was diligent in pursuing the people who had scammed us, stolen our money and our time, and left me in constant tears. Normally, I am a very relaxed, laid-back, and happy girl, but this had completely changed my demeanor. Nothing had ever affected me so. I was depressed.

In my mom's quest for justice, she met many other people who were scammed and who had left the training organization as hopeless and distraught as we were. During her communications with these other mothers, she met a lady who knew about a litter of newborn puppies in Florida. They were of Wildrose lineage, with both parents coming from Wildrose Kennels. This lady said that we could have our pick of one of the seven British Lab puppies when they turned seven weeks old. We could start over. I could train my own puppy.

How thankful I am for that dear lady! However, at the time I was not as thrilled as you would expect. I was still so discouraged by what had happened, and had lost all hope. I had convinced myself that there was no such thing as a diabetic alert dog. Having put my faith in the first dog, which was a disaster, I didn't want to do it again. Could I really train a dog all by myself? How would I know what to do? Did I really want to get a dog and spend all of my time teaching it simple things like "sit" and "down?" How did I know I could even housetrain this little puppy, much less train it to save my life? I didn't want to have anything to do with it.

On the other hand, people had donated so much money towards the purpose of getting me a diabetic alert dog. Was it right to just give up? My mom and I wrestled with this right up until the night before we left for Florida. At three in the morning, I finally decided that we would go. We got a few hours of sleep and then started out for Florida. Still conflicted, I had a nasty attitude on the way down there. "I'm coming, but not because I want to!"

My three younger siblings, Beth, Lydia, and Timothy, traveled on this twelve-hour journey with us. My mom and I took turns driving, and my dad stayed home to hold the fort down. That was one thing about the trip I was actually excited about: I got to drive. I had gotten my learner's permit the previous month and I was able to put my skills to the test on the way to Florida. Then, when we finally arrived, I actually started to get a little bit excited. I was anxious to see the puppies, but we visited with the owners first. Finally, they let us go out to see the puppies. Seven red and yellow little British Labs ran up to me with their tales wagging and their big ears flopping. They were more than enough to melt my heart.

One little puppy caught my attention more than all the others. I had planned to choose a girl, but this boy was amazing. He had just sneaked into the barn and he had started eating out of the bag of dog food, so he had a big round tummy. The darkest of the litter, his ears were the biggest and his tail wagged the most. He was spunky. I liked this one. I thought he liked me too. I thought it was amazing that this dog wagged his tail so much, something that I did not see with my other dog. This little puppy was happy, and it made me happy to see him happy. We played some games with all the puppies, but I kept my eyes out on this one little puppy that was wearing a little bitty red collar. I wanted him.

We hid a bowl of food to see if the puppies could use their noses to find it. The cute pup in the red collar that had stolen my heart in only seconds always found the food first. I picked him up and held him up to my chest. His tail started wagging and he looked up at my face and started licking my lips. That nasty fish breath didn't bother me. I loved him.

I got to take that cute little nasty-breath puppy home with me. We loaded up in the car and I held him in my lap. He was so soft and fuzzy. But this puppy had no name. I had not planned to fall in love with a puppy. I had planned to have a terrible attitude. I planned to take home a puppy only because it was the right thing to do, so I hadn't thought about any names. On the drive home my siblings were suggesting name ideas. My dad called me and told me to name him "Winston" or "Churchill." None of these names matched this cute little roly-poly in my arms.

It finally came to me: Mr Darcy! Yes, Mr Darcy! From my favorite book, *Pride and Prejudice*, Mr Darcy was the perfect name. And how fitting that name is! You see, in the book, Mr Darcy is always behind the scenes fixing everyone's problems. No one knows that Mr Darcy is the one who is making everything okay, but he is the one responsible for everything going the right way.

It was the perfect name for this cute little puppy who would one day be the one behind the scenes giving me the ability to sleep at night, to drive, to go to college, and to move out on my own! Today maybe people just see me doing all these things and think, "She is a strong girl," but that isn't why I can do what I do. Mr Darcy is the one who's behind the scenes keeping me healthy and making everything possible.

I took Mr Darcy home and spent every moment with him. Not at all used to having a little puppy with me, I didn't know exactly what to expect. I certainly made loads of mistakes, such as laying him on my bed right next to my backpack as I started to unpack my toiletries from our Florida trip. When I walked to the bathroom and came back, Mr Darcy had completely chewed through the cord of my hair dryer. I had no idea that I couldn't leave him there for three minutes. I had a lot to learn, and so did Mr Darcy. I took Mr Darcy outside to go to the bathroom every half hour at first. If I forgot to take him out that often, he would have an accident. I had to learn what to do when Mr Darcy would start chewing on the leash he was wearing. Mr Darcy took up every moment of every day. In the middle of the night, he would wake me up whining. We would go for a midnight walk together. I talked to him about everything. Even when he was sound asleep, I would tell him all about my diabetes and about my blood sugars. I would talk to him about how I felt, and about how I wish it wasn't time to change my insulin pump site. He was a good listener. If something sounded particularly interesting he would tilt his head and stare at me with his big brown eyes. I had only had this little puppy for a few days and he was already my best friend.

I did sacrifice a lot for my best friend, though. All of my time went to him. When I was invited to do something with friends, I could only accept the invitation if it was something that Mr Darcy, at his young age, could do with me. My mom said it was as if I had become a parent prematurely. Instead of just thinking about myself, I was forced to think about another living, breathing thing. Whenever we went out, I had to get myself ready, and then get Mr Darcy ready. My mom had sewn him a little vest that said, "Service Dog In Training. Please Don't Pet" and strapped it around his fat, puppy tummy. When he got bigger, he wore a full-blown vest that held all of my diabetes supplies: my meter, pricker, test strips, a juice box, an insulin pen, and a pump site change just in case. But when Mr Darcy was a little puppy and still learning, I had to carry a bag with all of Mr Darcy's supplies in it: a bottle of water, a bowl, treats, a bone, and wet wipes in case of an accident. Because I was homeschooled at the time, I could dedicate all day to Mr Darcy, even neglecting schoolwork for him. People have no idea the sacrifice it takes to make this work. Caring for and training Mr Darcy was a huge responsibility.

Every day we played games with the scent of my low blood sugar. Whenever I had a low blood sugar, my mom helped me spit on cotton swabs so we could freeze them. Those swabs would have the scent of my low blood sugar on them. Later we could hide those for Mr Darcy and train him to find the scent. I would have my mom keep Mr Darcy in the kitchen while I hid somewhere in the back of the house with the low scent hidden in my clothes. My mom would give Mr Darcy the command to "Go find Abi; find the low!" Mr Darcy would run through the halls, slipping and sliding all the way down. He would come find me and his little nose would sniff all over me until he found the target. When he found the low scent we would all jump up and scream in excitement for him. "Good boy! You found the low! Yay Mr Darcy! What a smart puppy!" We would shower him with pets, kisses, hugs, treats, and scratches on his butt (his favorite place to be scratched). When Mr Darcy found the low scent he would get all the fun, good, happy things that he loved the most.

We played games with the low scent for about two weeks with Mr Darcy. After that we would only play this "low game" with him when I was actually low. The game was the same except we would reward him when he found me and started smelling my breath, which gave off the low scent. When Mr Darcy found a low, the rest of life stopped. My sisters would stop studying, my brother would put down his Legos, my mom would leave the food in the kitchen, and my dad would come from his office just to tell Mr Darcy what a good boy he was. At the time we followed no research about diabetic-alert-dog training. I would do what made sense. If it worked, I would keep on doing it. We just made it fun for Mr Darcy.

One time, when he was nine weeks old, I was sitting on the kitchen floor and Mr Darcy ran up to me and started licking my face, profusely. Could it be that he was trying to tell me my blood sugar was low? Maybe, but maybe not. It couldn't hurt to test and see. We tested my blood sugar and found that it was low. It was 70 mg/dl (milligrams per deciliter). We were so proud of Mr Darcy. He had alerted to a low blood sugar level. He did it all by himself. I didn't give him a cue; he didn't need my help; I didn't even know that I was low. This was going to work after all!

As the weeks went on, Mr Darcy continued to alert to low

blood sugar just like he had done that very first day. He continued to come to me and lick my face when I was low. He got better and better as time passed, getting more consistent. He was amazing. By the time he was four months old he was alerting to low blood sugar episode that I had, even in the middle of the night. This was a miraculous answer to our thousands of prayers.

After he had shown he'd have no problems alerting to low blood sugars, he started alerting to my high blood sugars. He would bound up to me and kissed me a million miles a minute when he smelled that my blood sugar was high, just like he did when my blood sugar went low. This didn't take any extra training at all. He just started picking up on these episodes. He was so in tune with the smell of my body that he knew when something was wrong.

When Mr Darcy was six months, I thought I had a fully trained dog. I thought I was a perfect little dog trainer. Boy, was I wrong. At around that time my mom and I took Mr Darcy to Wildrose Kennels. In emails and on the phone, we had told the Stewarts at Wildrose all about Mr Darcy and how amazing he was. We told them how he was saving my life, even waking me up in the middle of the night. They were amazed by our stories.

When we arrived with Mr Darcy during a puppy-picking day, everyone circled around him as if he were some sort of movie star. People were staring at him in awe. When Mr Darcy caught a glimpse of the Stewart's lake, he was intrigued. He had never seen a lake before. He stared at it. Then, in just the moment it took for him to see a duck in the lake, Mr Darcy was gone in a flash. He jumped into the lake with his vest on and all. He swam out into the middle, grabbed the duck decoy, and brought it to me.

I had never been so embarrassed. Mr Darcy continued the tour of Wildrose soaking wet. He did okay, but he wasn't particularly impressive. Every now and then his nose would go to the ground and start sniffing everywhere. If he saw a duck across the lake, he would whine because he wanted to go get it.

Our trip to Wildrose showed me that Mr Darcy did have a few more things to learn about obedience. We went back to Wildrose many times after our first experience there. Sometimes at Wildrose, Mike Stewart would throw some ideas about obedience training my way. I would go home and work on the ideas he gave me. When we would go back to Wildrose again, Mr Mike would be proud of the way Mr Darcy had improved. But there was always more work to be done. Obedience training was much harder than scent training for Mr Darcy. Scent training was natural to him. He was bred to be a scenting dog. Obedience took more work for him. The hardest skill I would ever have to teach Mr Darcy was how to "heel." Mr Darcy needed to be able to walk alongside my knee at the same pace I was walking. He should never lag behind, and never pull ahead. He is a fast-paced, active dog and generally did not lag behind, but it was a struggle to teach him not to pull ahead of me. In my normal outing places like church, the grocery store, and the mall, Mr Darcy had the perfect heel. However, when we would go to a new and more distracting place, like Wildrose, Mr Darcy would walk way too fast. One time when we were at Wildrose, Mr. Mike invited Mr Darcy and me to go on a walk with him and one of his dogs. He showed me his methods of training a dog to heel. I watched, and later also tried out my own ideas. Teaching Mr Darcy to heel required all of my attention. I worked diligently on his training. Most of the time I loved it. He was a joy. Sometimes, though, it did get overwhelming. It was a lot of responsibility for a teenager to handle. Once, when we went to a Memorial Day Service where my dad was the speaker, I so wanted to listen to my dad speak, but I had to walk Mr Darcy around and around and around the park during the service so that he wouldn't whine. There would be guns going off after my dad finished speaking. I had to keep Mr Darcy occupied so that the guns wouldn't catch him off guard. Everyone else got to listen except for me. I would spend my whole day with Mr Darcy. I usually spent about an hour in the mornings outside with him working on heeling, sitting, lying down, waiting, and coming to me when I called him. I then would go inside and let him rest while I held his leash and did some reading. We would spend an hour or so working on tricks that he already knew, and I would constantly add new skills for him to learn. I would sometimes give him a treat while working on a new trick, but most of the time all Mr Darcy needed was a high pitched, happy "Good boy, Mr Darcy!" In the afternoon we would go outside and I would throw some tennis balls for him, and when he was older I taught him how to jump through hula hoops. I tried to find somewhere to take him in public every day, even if it was just the grocery store. In the evening we would work on staying in place on his mat and I would teach him not to get up. Training was a constant, all-day thing.

It was worth it, though. He would wake me up in the middle of the night because my blood sugar was low. I would drink a juice box and then hold him in my lap and squeeze him tightly and whisper into his big, soft ears, "Thank you, Buddy!" I would do anything for those moments. Those moments made turning down invitations to spend the night with a friend easy.

***

Mr Darcy loves being outside. He can stand out there with his head in the air, just sniffing for hours. He loves to run around with a tennis ball in his mouth, or just lie under a tree and let his ears fly back in the wind. It is torture for Mr Darcy to stay inside. It was often difficult to get him to even come inside.

Once, I had let Mr Darcy outside the kitchen door to use the bathroom. It was a beautiful, sunny day and the wind was blowing. It was the perfect weather for a dog to be playing outside. My mom called me into the living room to look at some pictures she had pulled up on the computer. She was sitting at the computer desk and I was standing, looking over her shoulder. All of a sudden we heard a shrill, sharp yelp. It sounded as if Mr Darcy had gotten hurt. Immediate panic swept over us. I was worried that a car had hit him. We ran into the kitchen and saw Mr Darcy standing on the other side of the glass door. He looked fine. I opened the door and he immediately ran in, jumped up, and started licking my face in a panic. My mom ran to the counter and grabbed my meter. She threw it to me, and I checked my blood sugar as fast as I possibly could. I was low. My blood sugar was 65 mg/dl. This is an amazing dog, I thought. He had smelled my blood sugar when he was outside and I was through the kitchen and in the living room. When Mr Darcy was about a year old and fabulous at alerting me for both high and low blood sugar, I decided to change the way he alerted. He had always licked my face to tell me that I was low or high. That had worked very well. However, I decided that maybe there would be something more appropriate in public than his jumping up on me and licking me. When he was a little, twelve-pound puppy it was cute and fun for him to climb up onto my lap and lick my face. Now that he was a forty-five-pound Lab, climbing on me and licking me was no longer cute or comfortable.

My mom and I learned about something called a bringsel from other dog trainers. The bringsel is a stick-shaped object that is soft, basically a cylinder of material stuffed with quilting foam. A lot of search and rescue dogs use bringsels in their work. I loved the idea of using this for Mr Darcy's alert. I started to train Mr Darcy to pick up the bringsel in his mouth and carry it to me when I was low or high. This was easy to train him to do. At first I would keep the bringsels put away where Mr Darcy could not see them or get to them. When he would come to me to alert to a low blood sugar, I would quickly get one of the bringsels out and give it to him as I said, "Here's the bringsel! Good low! Tell me with the bringsel! Good boy, Mr Darcy!" He would grab it as I petted him all over and rewarded him for alerting. Then I would take it from him and put it away until the next time my blood sugar went low. I would put the bringsels out of reach at first so that Mr Darcy would not just play with it. He needed to understand that the bringsel was serious. It was not a toy. After about two weeks of keeping the bringsels hidden and only getting them out when Mr Darcy had already alerted, I started putting the bringsels on a very low shelf in our kitchen.

One of the shelves was only about four inches off the ground, so Mr Darcy could easily reach the bringsel. If he came to alert to my low blood sugar and didn't have a bringsel I would say, "Let's go get a bringsel for this low!" and we would walk to the shelf. I would point to the bringsels and he would pick one up. Then, of course, we told Mr Darcy how good he was for getting a bringsel. Within a few days he would never come to me to alert to a low or high blood sugar without a bringsel in his mouth. It became natural for him. He loved carrying things in his mouth, and he picked up on alerting me with the bringsel. The bringsel also kept him from licking my face. Mr Darcy loved to take the bringsel to my other family members, too. When he took it to my mom, she would say, "Good low, Mr Darcy!" He was so proud of himself when he got to show off his cool trick to everyone who was in the house.

Mr Darcy still uses the bringsel, but now he knows how to distinguish between high and low blood sugar. He brings me the bringsel and waves it at me if I am low, and he bows in front of me if I am high. He was always eager to learn something new, and he already knew how to wave to me and bow in front of me on command. It was simple to tie these tricks into his alerts.

Mr Darcy truly is an amazing dog, but that isn't to say that he hasn't gotten into his share of trouble. He was bitten by a snake and sprayed with pepper spray. He swallowed string that could have killed him, hurt his leg, had stitches put into his tail, got lost, threw up in Wal-Mart, and was attacked by another dog.

Are all dogs this unlucky? You just never know what's going to happen when you're dealing with Mr Darcy.

Mr Darcy is way too smart for his own good. He knows how to open every door in my house. He even knows how to open cabinets. He can smell a tennis ball from a mile away.

When he was four months old he figured out how to open the Rubbermaid container that held his food. Once I left him in my room for no more than ten minutes. When I came back, Mr Darcy had opened the latch, propped the lid up, and had eaten half of his bucket of food. I found him with his mouth full of food, his front legs hanging over the food bucket, and looking as fat and as happy as ever.

***

When I was sixteen and Mr Darcy was a little over one year old, we went to Itawamba Community College. I was enrolled on the Tupelo campus, which was about 45 minutes from where my parents and I lived. Mr Darcy came with me every day. He became the unofficial college mascot. Everyone there knew him and loved him. He was so popular that I decided to make him his own Facebook page where I could share stories about him, pictures of him, and videos of him. It took less than a week for Mr Darcy to have far more fans than I have friends.

While at school, Mr Darcy would quietly lie under my desk in each of my classes. Despite the fact that others could see a big, sixty-pound, red dog in the classroom, they couldn't even notice that he was there. He stayed quiet and still. That is, unless my blood sugar went high or low. When my blood sugar would drop or rise, Mr Darcy would crawl out from under the desk, grab the bringsel that was attached to his leash, and climb into my lap so I could get my meter out of his vest. He was wonderful. Because of him, I never had to leave a classroom, miss a lecture, or turn in a late homework assignment. He would always alert before my blood sugar got dangerously low so that I could just drink a juice box as I was in class. He made college with diabetes a possibility for me.

One day I was in one of my classes and there was a fly buzzing around. It would fly around my fellow students' heads, they would swat it off, and then it would go find someone else to annoy. We were all watching the fly intently so that we would be prepared to swat it off whenever it came near. As it continued to fly around students' heads, they swatted it, and it flew down towards the floor. Then the stupid fly made a terrible choice. It flew around Mr Darcy's head. Mr Darcy quietly, and without ever getting up from his comfy spot under my desk, opened his mouth, caught the fly, and swallowed it. When he licked his chops with his big red tongue, the entire classroom burst into laughter, even the professor.

Not only did Mr Darcy help me while I was in classes, but he also helped me on my way to classes. On the 45-minute drive to school, Mr Darcy was my copilot. He always sat in the passenger seat while I was driving. He looked so regal, sitting tall in the front seat looking out the window. Several times on our drive I saw him pick up his bringsel and look at me. I remember pulling over, testing my blood sugar, and drinking a juice box. I would call my mom to tell her what had happened and that I might be home a little bit late. What a miracle! I could have had a seizure on the road while driving. I could have killed myself or other people, but Mr Darcy kept me safe.

After a year of attending school at the community college, I got a job there, working as a secretary for financial aid. Needless to say, Mr Darcy worked there, too. The staff loved him. He was very well known around the school. There was, of course, the occasional student who would think that I was blind, or see Mr Darcy and run away screaming in fear, but I just had to laugh and move on.

Sometimes, however, it is not a laughing matter. I remember

one time at school, I was standing at the counter taking care of my tuition fees. I was waiting in line when I heard someone across the room barking. A guy was standing across the room, looking at Mr Darcy and barking at him. I decided to be mature about it and ignore the situation. I continued through the line and then took care of my business. As I started to leave, the man started barking even louder. I could not ignore this. I turned around and said, "Um, sir, are you barking at my dog? Because I think if my dog is well-behaved enough to not bark in a public establishment, you can be that well-behaved, too!"

Having a service dog also means standing up for my rights. I often encounter people who are ignorant of the public access laws concerning disabilities and service dogs. Let me just say, it is not "cool" to have to argue your way into Wal-Mart when you're with a group of friends only to get in the store and have every employee and customer stare at you, point at you, and whisper behind your back.

Once I was in a store looking at the musical Hallmark cards. I noticed two elderly ladies standing at the end of the aisle. One of them was pointing at me as she whispered, "Did you see that blind girl?"

The other lady whispered back, "Oh, Sweetie, I don't think she's blind. She's probably deaf!"

So having a service dog is hard. How do I stand up for my rights without being disrespectful? How do I politely tell someone who is older than me to stop petting my dog? There are a lot of hard things to balance. The alerting is what makes it all worth it, but even alerting brings challenges.

For example, one day I was having what I call a "bad diabetes day." I was having low blood sugar after low blood sugar after low blood sugar. Mr Darcy would alert and I would test. I would be low, and I would drink juice or eat a snack. Then in fifteen minutes Mr Darcy would come back, alert, I would test, I would still be low, and then I would eat again. It happened again and again. I had had at least eleven lows that day. I had drunk so much juice, and had eaten countless packages of peanut butter crackers. I was physically and emotionally exhausted. I was tired, and I was tired of diabetes. I was doing everything right, and yet I was still low. I had eaten over one hundred and twenty carbs and I had even suspended my pump so that I would not be getting insulin—and I was still low! Sitting on the sofa resting, overwhelmed, and holding back the tears, I saw the last thing I wanted to see: Mr Darcy walking in with the bringsel. When he came through the door, I broke down and started crying, "Please, don't alert! I don't want another alert! I'm sick of being low! Make it stop!"

Mr Darcy was doing his job, yet I was mad at him. I didn't want to reward him for doing what was good. I didn't want to act proud of him and act happy for him that he had alerted to a low, because I didn't want to be low. But I have to reward him.

I let Mr Darcy continue swimming with my sister and my husband, Jordan Atkinson. He was swimming calmly alongside my husband when I saw him suddenly turn around, stick his nose up in the air, and start sniffing. He started frantically swimming towards the dock. I thought he had run out of breath or gotten tired and was panicking. He made it to the dock very quickly and climbed up the ladder all by himself. When he got up he ran to me and grabbed my meter case. I checked my blood sugar and I was high. As it turns out, my pump had fallen off and I didn't know it. I wasn't getting insulin and I would have kept on getting higher and higher if Mr Darcy had not alerted me.

Now Mr Darcy goes to school with me at the University of Alabama. He no longer brings the bringsel to my parents and my siblings to tell them that my blood sugar is high or low. Now he brings it to my husband. He still makes me laugh, and he still makes me cry. He still gets into trouble, and I still sometimes find myself in the office of an emergency veterinarian. I still make sacrifices for him and he still alerts for me. He still wakes me up in the middle of the night. He still brings me my meter in the middle of the day.

Mr Darcy has been with me through changing schools, moving to a new house in a new state, and getting married, Mr Darcy continues to do his job and he loves every minute of it. Still, after all of the trials, had I known how hard it would be to have a service dog before I got into this, I am completely positive that I still would have chosen that fuzzy, little bitty, red-collared, stinky-breath puppy, Mr Darcy.

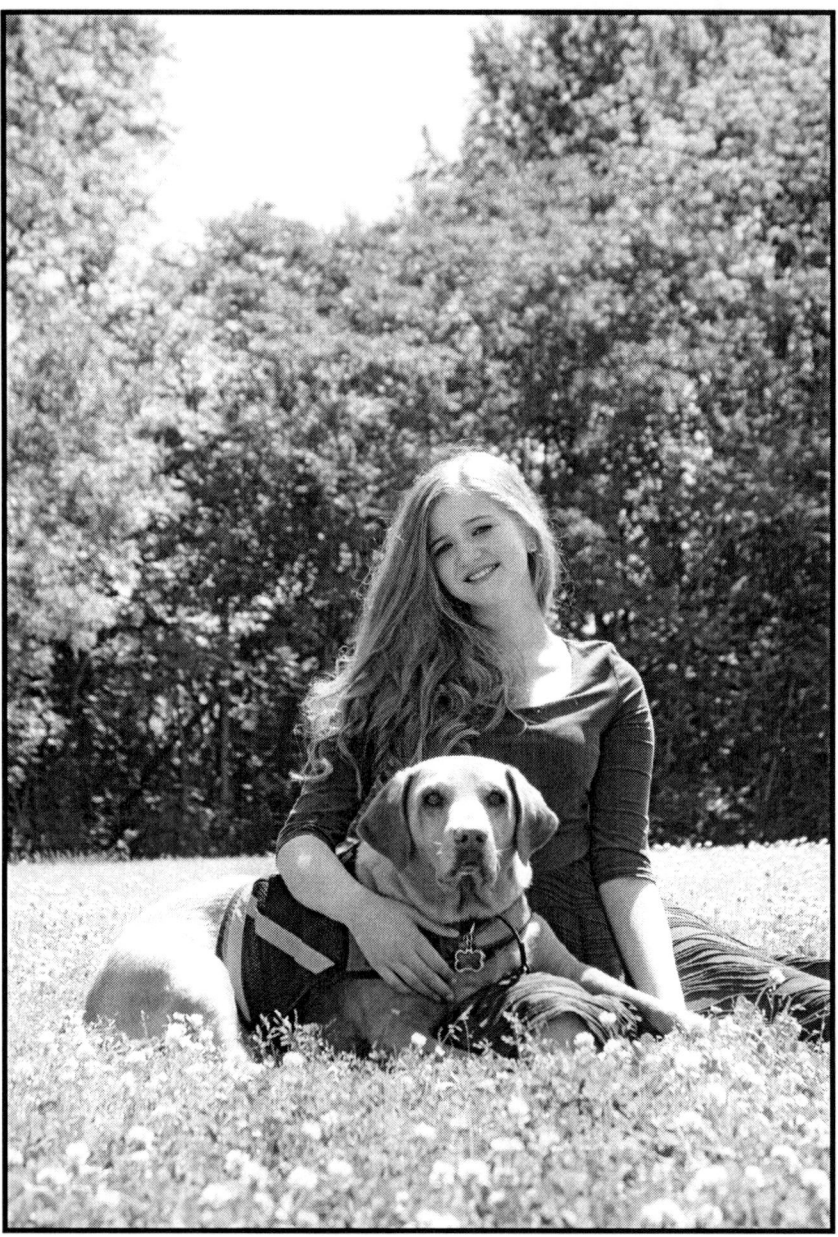

Teddy Bear with Ciara Smith.

Teddy Bear and Capri and Ciara Smith: Communal Knowledge

MY LEGS FELT LIKE JELLY. I tried to coordinate their movements, but my brain was firing erratically, and I couldn't seem to get the correct messages telegraphed to my feet. I moved along the corridor riding a nightmare. The green tiles from the walls, cold and hard, floated into my eyesight. It was surreal. This couldn't be my life, and that couldn't be my daughter being rushed down the hall on a gurney with a nurse squeezing the air bag, manually filling Ciara's lungs, forcing air into her unresponsive body. My leg slipped out, and I went down hard on my knee, my crutches clattering out beside me. Up again, scrabbling, run-hobbling down that corridor.

The day had started like every day since my baby, Ciara, was diagnosed at six years of age with type 1 diabetes. I woke her up for blood checks and shots. She was far better about the shots than I was. It took long minutes standing there with the syringe in my hand, poised to jab her skin and deliver the life-saving insulin dose. I had to breathe deeply. I had to project a calm that I did not feel in order to get my hand to stop shaking, so that I could give the shot without bending the needle against

Ciara's delicate skin. I was the kind of mom who had to leave the doctor's office during my children's immunization shots to sob in the hallway. I couldn't stand the thought of my kids getting pricked by needles. Now here I was, a mom required to give shots a minimum of seven times a day. I had to prick Ciara's finger and squeeze out the blood droplet to test her blood sugar (BG) levels an average of twenty times a day. I had to. This was our life now that Ciara was diagnosed. Ciara was far braver than I was.

✳✳✳

When we got up this particular morning, we thought this was going to be a happy day. There was a little girl with type 1 diabetes who lived in our area and was just Ciara's age. They were going to meet in the afternoon for a play date. Ciara's blood sugar numbers had been fairly stable that day, by some miracle. We went to buy flowers for the girl's family. When we got back in the car, I checked Ciara's BG. She was a safe 132. A normal blood sugar number is around 100, and we aimed to keep Ciara within the 70-180 range. I was in the habit of checking her constantly. Ciara's blood sugar could shift in polar and unpredictable ways. Her numbers could shoot up into the 300s and then drop down to 27 in a matter of minutes. And that meant she would have a seizure. Constant vigilance. Constant checking. 132 was good, though. It was the same number as when we had left the house.

I started to drive home, but my mommy-radar had been humming in my head and was picking up its volume. "Danger! Danger!" I listened. It was the same radar call that I had heard the morning when I knew Ciara was going to die, raced her to the doctor, and she was diagnosed with type 1 diabetes. It was a primal limbic call-to-action. I stopped the car and checked Ciara's blood again. 132. I used my cell phone to get in touch with our endocrinologist. "Is it possible for a meter to be off?

Something's wrong with Ciara, and it's reading 132." My voice must have comported my conviction because he sent me straight to the hospital.

I buzzed past my neighborhood without any regard for the speed limit. My lights were on high; my hazards were flashing; I leaned on my horn. I drove to save my daughter's life, sometimes on the shoulder of the road, blasting past slower-moving cars, praying for safety, praying for everyone to get out of my way. Praying that I didn't crash, because Ciara wouldn't survive it. My foot jumped and shook on the gas pedal, so I stamped it down to the floor for control and barreled our jacked-up Land Cruiser down the highway. I called the hospital. Be ready! In the back seat, Ciara was screaming and seizing.

I came off the exit to the hospital. The emergency room and help was there on the right. I was so close, when a white car stopped in front of me. Like a deer-in-the-headlights, they seemed unable to move. Trees blocked me from driving around. I blared my horn with urgency. Nothing. I jumped out of the truck and screamed at the top of my lungs. I was on crutches from having my knee rebuilt and even though Ciara was only thirty-two pounds, I couldn't lift her and walk. Another driver appeared. He had the door open; he was untangling Ciara from the mess of seatbelt that had cocooned her while she was seizing. Now she was white-lipped and wilted, unconscious in this stranger's arms. He held her with such tenderness, as if she were a rare and delicate bloom that he was afraid he might bruise. I touched his sleeve, "Please, sir, can you run?" And he ran.

I followed the man as best I could into the hospital. The doctors checked her BG right away—still 132. They had no idea what to do. They watched as Ciara pulled into the fetal position, and her hands curled in. I knew what I was watching. I had read about this many times in my graduate studies at a Virginia medical college. My daughter was dying. She was going to die.

This was her last day. These were her last minutes. And I was powerless. Completely powerless.

The next few minutes were the building blocks of hell. Ciara stopped breathing, and they intubated her; they got her heart going again with chest compressions. They strapped her to the gurney and raced her down the corridor to God-knows-where. And I gave chase, pitching myself forward on my crutches, because in my fevered brain I thought that having my eyes on my baby girl gave her weight, increased the hold of gravity, tethered Ciara to her body and this world, and I would be able to keep her—she wouldn't leave me. She couldn't leave me.

Diabetes is Hell. It's a war. It's battle after battle. Rest and rise to fight again. I never knew this before Ciara was diagnosed. Like most people, I thought that it was a matter of management. Take your medicine, eat healthy foods, exercise, and everything would be just fine. It was not just fine. It was everything *but* just fine. I don't think there exists the right vocabulary to convey how "not fine" things were in Ciara's world.

✳✳✳

To explain, let me take you back a month earlier to Ciara's diagnosis. It was a holiday weekend, Labor Day. We were in the hospital for three days, and only saw an emergency room doctor. Ciara went a whole day—eleven hours—with no food, because the doctors would not give an insulin dose order to the nurses. And no amount of my browbeating was helping. I was labeled a pain in the neck. I labeled myself my child's advocate.

Because they never arrived, I gave up on the endocrine group that had come recommended to me. We were completely frustrated with the level of care Ciara was receiving. Our pediatrician found another doctor—a former Harvard pediatric endocrine professor—who was willing to take on Ciara's case. He told us to get her out of the hospital; she would be safer at home. Before we were discharged, my husband and I got a half-hour diabetes lesson. We learned how to draw up a shot and how to administer it. How to check blood sugar levels, but not what they meant. "Here's a stuffed bear to practice on," the diabetic educator said, smiling, as she shoved it into a canvas bag with a children's book and an adult's book and a "Good luck!" No one mentioned seizures. No one mentioned comas. No one mentioned that the nurse was really packing up our heaver sack, inadequately supplied, for the battles ahead.

Ciara felt awful after we left the hospital. "Mommy, if you love me, you'll take me to the doctor's," she would beg, cupping my chin in her little hands. And every day we went to the doctor. We went to the pediatrician; we went to the endocrinologist. We sat in their offices for hours on end so Ciara could be observed. But they did nothing to make her feel better. My husband, Todd, and I farmed out our other children—Blythe, Devin, and Aiden—to neighbors and friends, people who rallied behind us and made sure that if nothing else I could rest assured that my other three kids were fed and safe.

Something was going very badly with Ciara's blood sugar numbers. They were swinging wildly. The doctor surmised that I was doing something radically wrong. He sent a nurse to observe me for twelve hours. I realized while the nurse was there that she was hawk-eyed about every move I made when I was near Ciara. I realized that she was watching me to see if I was a candidate for a Münchausen by proxy diagnosis. Had a blood test existed for how I felt inside, as if I were constantly going over the top of a very high roller coaster, as if I were in a free fall and grabbing desperately at the slick sides of nothing for a handhold or a toehold or anything that felt like stability, they would not have been watching me, but would have been doing more tests on Ciara. The nurse passed me with flying colors, but was unable to figure out why Ciara's blood sugar numbers created the structure for that roller coaster that we rode without cease. Up and down. Up and down.

These violent swings caused Ciara to have seizures. Seizures manifested in different ways on different days. She could suddenly go blind and walk into trees and walls. Her face and body were covered in bruises. Bruises that made strangers give me hard and angry looks when we were out in public. The seizures collapsed Ciara in stores, where her legs and arms kicked out; her eyes rolled back in her head, and she lost control of her bladder. They caused her to think that I was the devil who was trying to poison her, as I tried to force the life-saving glucose gel into her mouth and down her throat. She would fight for her life as adrenaline gave power to muscles that defended her endangered brain. She kicked at my injured knee; she grabbed handfuls of hair and ripped them from my head; she beat against me with her fists. I looked every bit as battle-worn as she did. We looked abused. Diabetes was abusing us.

Diabetes requires pinpoint accuracy and regimentation. My family culture, however, was not geometrically built. I was more of a free-flow, amorphous kind of mom. I secularly home-schooled my children because I wanted us to be able to lie around, cuddled up in blankets with hot cocoa, and read books aloud all day. I served my kids organic vegetarian foods, and since they never had huge appetites and preferred to graze throughout the day, that's what we did.

My first marching orders from our new doctor concerned food.

Ciara had to eat at specific times, precisely at nine in the morning, noon, three, six and eight in the afternoon. On the dot. Not a minute before and not a minute after. She had thirty minutes to eat her meals. So my gregarious, storytelling daughter, who loved to sit and chat over dinner, had to put her head in her plate and shovel food. My vegetarian, grazing family now sat down to military precision and beef. I spent a long time with cookbooks and websites building a perfect menu for Ciara.

She had to love each thing because I could no longer say, "A picky child is a hungry child." My child would never have the luxury of being hungry, of not eating, of turning up her nose at something she didn't like. She would eat exactly what was on her plate, no more, no less and in thirty minutes flat. We did this to remove one more variable from the list of what could possibly be going wrong. But it didn't seem to help.

Now our food ways were changed and our days were filled with new diabetes components. Our family became structured. We were precise. We were careful. We were vigilant. We were consumed. But it didn't make Ciara feel better. All of our efforts didn't make her safer. Nothing I had tried worked. She kept getting sick. It was in prayerful meditation one night, waiting for the nurse to come for Ciara's every half-hour blood check, that I heard an answer in my head. *Ciara needs a service dog,* I thought. An answer so clearly spoken, and so resounding in conviction, that it could not be mistaken for anything but *the* answer to my prayer. I had been expressing my gratitude for knowing to take Ciara to the hospital, and I was thinking about what my clue had been that she was in imminent danger. I remembered the strange smell on the very top of Ciara's head—like the freshly wet diaper of a newborn. And the thought came to me: *If I can smell it, surely a dog can smell it long before. If a dog can smell it long before, and I can intervene faster, Ciara will be safe.* And that was it, my lighthouse in the dismally thick swirl of diabetes fog. As we bobbed up and down on the turbulent swells of the next two years, I clung to the raft of hope, and I aimed steadfastly in the direction of our beacon, a service dog.

We drove back home from the hospital on a Friday. It was good to be back in my own bed. It was raining in torrents throughout the night and the next day, bending the trees and causing blackouts. I was so grateful because this was the day of the Juvenile Diabetes Fundraising Walk, and now I didn't feel guilty for not going. I had already given everything I had to diabetes. I just wanted to cozy up with my family and breathe.

Life returned to the same battlefield we had left. Ciara suffered from violent blood sugar swings. She had frequent seizures. There was a change in our diabetic care: the hospital pediatric care doctors felt that Ciara would be better off using an insulin delivery pump. No more shots. Thank goodness! We had looked into other known technologies as well. There is such a thing as a continuous glucose monitor (CGM), for example, but Ciara's swings happened so quickly that the half-hour delay on a CGM reading made it ineffective. I knew that a trained service dog would be able to smell the shifting sugar levels before they showed up on a meter or a monitor. After all, dogs can smell tiny cancer cells; surely a dog could smell something as systemically broad as sugar swings.

My quest to find an alert dog was unrelenting—and frustrating. The dogs were very expensive—if you could even find one.

Through my research I found a man in California who was working with diabetic alert dogs (DADs), but his clients had to live within an hour's drive. I considered moving. My letters to him went unanswered. I found a woman in Australia who did not require her clients to live within arm's reach and I wrote to her. I would take Ciara to Australia for a dog if needed. She wrote back that there was an organization in the United States and suggested that I try them before I flew halfway around the world.

Finally, I hit pay dirt. There was a charitable group in the Midwest that placed DADs. I wrote immediately, filled out their forms, sent my application fee, crossed my fingers, and held my breath. There was nothing negative out there about this group. Its reputation glowed. Miss America endorsed the group and PBS had done a special about service dogs spotlighting this group, as had *Good Morning America* and CNN. August, 2007, almost a year to the day of Ciara's diagnosis, I got a phone call from the Missouri representative telling me that Ciara had been accepted into their program, and because of the emergency state of Ciara's health, they had made an extra place in their next training group scheduled for February. I blubbered into the phone. I cried so hard that I couldn't stand. Crying came easily to me those days; my emotions were at the surface of my skin. But this was an emotion I had not experienced in a year's time. This was relief. My daughter was going to be safe! The scattered puzzle pieces of our world were going to fit back together. My mind whirled at the enormity of this. The motherly warm voice on the other end was kindness personified. She soothed me. She understood. Help was here. It was all going to be okay now.

***

Each alert dog would be chosen with thoughtful precision for its diabetic teammate by temperament and accuracy of alerts on the scent samples that we shipped overnight, packed carefully in dry ice, to the trainers. The trainers would spend many hours reviewing our family dynamic from the videotapes that we had sent in—training our dog to fit in seamlessly. Our dog would be able to alert to day and night high blood sugar numbers, low blood sugar numbers, and ketones. Should Ciara start to go low, the dog would open the fridge and bring her a juice box. We took video of our fridge so that our dog could be specifically trained for this. Should Ciara have blood sugar issues at night, the dog had been taught to press an alarm to wake us up. The dogs of older children and adults would be taught to use a special phone that dials 911 in case of emergency and to bark for help. Since Ciara was only seven, her dog would be trained for this later. I printed all of the documentation, and read the contract. It was all very benign. I needed to raise $7,000 by November. I have tried to raise money for various charities in the past; I had even done marketing for the symphony. Raising large amounts of money like this, especially in such a small window of time, is difficult.

I love to help. Being a part of a solution feels deep-down good inside of me. It brings me joy and satisfaction. I knew, as I started fund-raising that I was giving others the opportunity to have these feel-good emotions. It should have been a win-win-win. Ciara would get a safety dog, the organization would get the needed funding, and I would give others the opportunity to earn good-karma points. I knew my friends had felt badly that there was nothing that they could do to help. Now there was a tangible way to help.

Yet begging for my daughter's safety was an enormously stressful, horrible experience. It made me feel ineffectual, incapable, and desperate. Truth be told, at that point, that's how I was already feeling. I hated that this process put it in my face.

I was humbled by the generosity, time, and kindness of our friends. The story of my daughter's best friend, Maggie, still squeezes my heart. For her birthday, Maggie asked that no one bring her a gift, but instead bring a check to help her friend be safe. Through her efforts, and the efforts of her family, they raised a quarter of the money we needed. The happily wagging tail would be their contribution.

Just after we sent in the last of the checks, Ciara had a massive seizure. She was sleeping in bed next to me, so I could check her every hour. Ciara was having a dropsy night with lots of lows. I must have fallen asleep as the sun was coming up. All of a sudden, Ciara sat up beside me and made a wild noise and flopped back down. Her BG was 40, well below the 57 mark where the brain stops functioning properly. I had no idea how long I had slept. I had no idea how long she had been that low. I called to my husband, Todd, for help. Ciara's muscles were doing a macabre dance. She vomited and lost control of her bladder. She was screaming screams that made the hair stand off my head. I had squirted the gel. I had given the emergency Glucagon shot. I had sent Todd downstairs to call 911. As fear crawled up his throat, choking off his ability to speak, or act, or think, I screamed the information down the stairs, hoping that the operator could hear me and would send the paramedics to help us.

The rescue crew gathered in my bedroom. They knew our house; they knew our dogs' names; I recognized all of their faces as they gathered around Ciara. I stroked her arm and chanted, "Your dog is coming. Your dog is coming. Soon you will be safe, baby. Soon this will all be over," I lied to her. I hoped that there would be a service dog helping us soon, but the voice in my head told me that I was lying to Ciara, my family, and myself.

Once we sent all of the money to the Missouri organization, I no longer got to talk to the warm motherly voice. She had been fired. The voice that was on the phone now had a metallic quality to it. New contracts were sent. These were bizarre contracts that did not resemble the kind, nurturing wording of the contracts we had originally signed. We would be in Missouri for three weeks of training in February. We could be released from the program at any time, at the discretion of the director, with no recourse, no monies returned, and no dog. It wasn't even going to be our dog. The organization would maintain ownership of the dog, and we would have to return each year to re-certify. If we failed to re-certify, the dog could be removed from our home. Actually, at the discretion of the director, our dog could be taken from us at any point—for any reason. What? I *never* would have agreed to such unilateral and undefined terms and conditions.

These contracts must be signed or our place would be given to another diabetic. Of course, the donated money was given to the organization, as is required when donating to a charity. The money was not for Ciara's dog, it was to support the organization as a whole, and donators could not request their money back. Todd and I signed the contracts even though I knew they were bizarre and the lack of recourse made them illegal. I knew that this was not going to turn out well. My hands were stuck in the tar-baby fraud, and all I could do was hope that my inner voice was wrong.

In February, I packed the car and slipped and slid for two days through an ice storm to Missouri. Ciara and I were off on our adventure: Ciara joyful in the back of our pale-blue minivan, me gripping the wheel with all of my strength, the tension radiating down my spine.

I have to admit that I harbored a flicker of hope all the way up to the point that I walked into the motel lobby. Right away I recognized the director, Michelle: she was hard to miss and hard to mistake. I had seen her in the PBS special that we had borrowed from the library and on various public appearances on TV. Michelle was squat and round. Her kinky, long brown hair, streaked in grey, stood out triangularly from head to hip, as if she were a figure from a Diagon Alley scene in the *Harry Potter* movies. There she sat, holding court.

Ciara and I walked in, and I offered her a tentative smile. Michelle looked through us. She didn't seem to recognize us though we had sent the obligatory photos and videotapes of our family, our home, and our life. She had all of the ammunition that she would need to attack and belittle us for the next three weeks. But in this moment, she seemed to dismiss our existence. Ciara and I went to our temporary home to unpack our things. We encamped for our next battle—a battle of wills.

✳✳✳

On the very first day of "training," Ciara received her dog, Bo. He was a beautiful golden retriever. Ciara fell to the floor with a scream of bliss. She and Bo rolled around in giddy harmony. Bo was to be her lifeline, and Ciara loved him the second she saw him. Too bad Bo was crazy. Too bad the woman in charge of this swindle was even crazier. I remember day two of our "training" when the scam artist stood in front of my child and explained to me and the whole class that the reason Bo would never work for us was because I was an anxiety junkie, that my husband would divorce me so he could be with an attractive woman, and that my teens would commit suicide. Navigating this three-week-long labyrinth was going to be one of my life's big challenges.

Every day we gathered—dogs, children, parents, and staff—at the YMCA. Every day we went over puppy 101 lessons with four-year-old dogs. We learned how to walk a dog in a circle. Long hours were spent walking around and around and around. The dogs had poor heeling skills and all of them had prong collars to help manhandle them into obedience. We were given bandanas to hide this from the public, since the public wouldn't like the idea of a service dog so poorly trained that it required a pronged collar.

Along with the bandanas, we were given strange rules that were to be followed to the letter. We had to always carry baby powder with us, for example. No, I didn't know why, and I wasn't going to ask. By the woman's law, only the children could handle the dogs—ever. One of the most onerous rules was that the children had to potty the dogs for fifteen minutes, every two hours, or whenever we changed from one location to another. Even if the dogs had gone potty, it had to last fifteen minutes. Even if there was an ice storm, it had to be fifteen minutes. Even if it was midnight. Even if the kids had fevers and runny noses. This was non-negotiable. We were watched through windows and timed. We were caught on the motel security camera tapes trying to cheat the fifteen-minute rule. We parents were videotaped trying to let our children stand in the shelter of the building instead of in the ice-covered field. Our disobedience was brought up in the classroom. We were berated. If we continued to be defiant, our dogs would be removed, and we would be sent home.

It wasn't an idle threat. We knew that one child had been sent home in the middle of the last session. It was the little girl's tenth birthday, and she had been told that they were going to have a party for her with cake. As the little girl went into the conference room full of expectation and cheer, the woman snatched the dog's lead from the little girl's hand and told her to leave—she would not get a dog. The family's motel room had been cancelled, and they found themselves with no dog, nowhere to stay, and no hope. We were all shocked and horrified. This story was told to us with a twinkle in the woman's eye. She obviously found great joy in our reactions. This story kept us in line.

The woman had a whole bag of tricks to keep us in line. She sent us letters at the motel that told us that our placement in the program was fragile. These letters arrived at three in the morning, shoved under our door with scrape and a whoosh. I was awake to hear ours arrive; I couldn't sleep between my rattling nerves and Ciara's blood checks.

When we weren't working the dogs at the YMCA, we met at the local mall. Here we did strange things repetitiously for the three weeks. We walked up and down the stairs; we walked in and around the stores; we put the dogs in a down-stay under the benches. Okay, that all seemed reasonable. But we also had to stand next to our dogs while the staff ran up on them with shopping carts, stepped over and on them, hid around corners, and loudly dropped clipboards behind the dogs as we walked by—this was supposed to cure them of a startle response. It didn't cure me of my startle response, that's for sure. Bo would jump into the planters and hide under the shiny leaves of the devil's ivy.

Into the third week of our stay, we started doing the scent training. Prior to our coming, during the time at home when we had gathered the mandatory funds, we had also been gathering socks that our children had worn when they had a low blood sugar event. These socks were put in plastic baggies and frozen.

Once we had accumulated a dozen or so, we sent them, packed in dry ice to preserve the integrity of the low scent, overnight, to the dog trainers. The dogs were being trained for our individual child, we were told. Once we were there, however, we discovered that the sock bags had never been opened.

Scent training consisted of two components. First, we took a Pup-Peroni and put it in one of the socks that we had sent to the trainers. The sock was then placed under a plastic cup. The dog would have to indicate which of the three plastic cups in front of him held the sock with the Pup-Peroni. That was scent training. The second component was to hold up a clipboard with a piece of tape on it. We rubbed the tape with the Pup-Peroni and when the dog touched the tape, he was rewarded with a treat. Yes, it did seem random and absurd; no, it never progressed to a useful behavior.

Not only were these dogs not trained, they were also not healthy. One of them had a broken tail. They all had psychological disorders. Bo got motion sick and vomited in my car every time we drove. The dogs growled, barked, and nipped at our kids. It was our fault, of course: children should not run, children should not play, children should sit still, and in our case my child should not speak to any other child. Ciara was barred from interacting with anyone. The other families were warned against any contact with us. We were a contagion—they would catch the kicked-out-of-the-program disease from us. We were isolated.

Though our children were made the scapegoat for the dogs' poor behavior, our children's behavior could not explain the worms. The dogs had worms and took medicine to rid them of the parasites. These dogs were supposed to sleep with our children. I needed more information about the whole de-worming process, but I didn't ask. I didn't do anything that made it look like I was challenging authority. I made sure that Bo and Ciara didn't sleep together—and I made sure that the curtains in our first story room were always tightly drawn shut, so no one could spy on us and no one would know that I didn't allow a wormy dog to sleep with my child.

My husband had come up with a plan. If we were kicked out, I was to call him. He would fly out to meet us. He would drive us home. I was obviously too distressed to attempt the drive on my own. He had friends lined up to take in our other kids. Our retreat plans were in place.

Ciara, Bo, and I somehow made it through our three weeks of emotional abuse. We headed back to Virginia. I was immediately on the phone with trainers. I worked long hours, every day, from March until June, training Bo to be stable. I spent money we didn't have getting specialists to intervene. Long story short, the professionals all said what I already knew: Bo could not now, nor could he ever, function as anything other than a pet.

***

A young teen, Mark Rinkel, whose brother, Jason, had been in our class, won a prize for philanthropy. His prize money was to fund his charitable efforts. He started an organization called Red Alert with the mission of getting functioning DADs to families in need. Red Alert was named for the Rinkels' new dog, Red, who was being trained to work for Jason. Red was the offspring of a breeding pair of British Labs from Wildrose Kennels. Wildrose specializes in pure lines of British Labs, keen hunting dogs with wonderful dispositions. This breeding pair now lived in Florida, and had just produced a litter. Through Mark's efforts and the efforts of a few of the other moms, a service dog trainer evaluated the new pups. Four puppies were chosen as having the right traits for our needs. We were overjoyed that Mark provided our family with one of these puppies. The Thorntons got one as well.

On the day that we drove to Washington, D.C. to pick up our new puppy, we drove Bo to a friend's house. That family would foster Bo while he was being litigated in the courts. We needed

Bo to be away from the new puppy; we couldn't let him teach the puppy his crazy ways. Bo now happily hunts rocks at the bottom of the river and hikes with his boy. He leads a nap-filled life with no one asking anything from him other than to be a pet. Ciara was very sad, but very mature for a just-turned-eight-year-old, about having to give up Bo. Could it really only be June? Instead of four months, it seemed as if years had gone by since we had started out on the disastrous road to the Midwest.

Our two-hour drive to Washington to pick up our new-with-possibilities puppy did not have a festive quality. Ciara and I were quiet. There was no jubilation. We talked about possible names. We knew that our friend Abi Thornton had decided to name her puppy Mr Darcy, after a character in *Pride and Prejudice*, a favorite novel of mine. I pushed hard for Ciara to name her pup "Bingley," Mr Darcy's best friend in the book. My whole family booed the idea. But I still loved the name. Ciara had decided on "Frisby." That's a pretty good dog name, too.

As we parked the car and walked towards the airport to meet the new puppy, we held hands, and we held our breath. I think we both were defending ourselves against the next disappointment. But who could be disappointed when we walked up to the baggage pick-up area and there, in the little mauve crate, sat a strawberry-blonde ball of fur, with a little pink tongue, and a furiously wagging tail? I tried to focus on the sweetness of this little puppy and ignore the bitterness that still lingered at the back of my tongue. The name Frisby sailed out the door. This was cuddly, sweet, soft-bellied, warm Teddy Bear. This was Teddy Bear whose soft eyes could subdue the clouds and make us feel sunny again.

I drove home hearing giggling in the back seat as Teddy wrestled, licked, and unconditionally loved Ciara. I let her feel joy, while I did the worrying. I thought, *Now what do I do?* When we got home, I handed the puppy over to my older teens for a month: their job was to expose Teddy Bear to every sight, sound, and smell they could think of. Teddy went to train stations, horse farms, and Wal-Mart. Teddy smelled baby diapers, perfumes at Macy's, and hospitals. Teddy had umbrellas opened beside him, wheelchairs rolled towards him, and he listened to gunfire and cannons explode as he sat in a field. After our experience with terrified Bo, this puppy needed to become rock solid, or, in horse parlance, "bomb-proof."

After the month with my teens, Teddy Bear accompanied Ciara and me as we set off on another cross-country adventure. We were heading to Texas to meet with the other families who had banded together after the nightmare experience.

It was the beginning of July 2008, and Ciara, Teddy Bear, and I were on the road in No-Wheres, Texas, aiming north on the last leg of a three-day drive. There on the side of the road, with no cell phone bars and no other travelers to offer help, in 105-degree weather, Ciara had a massive seizure that lasted two hours. I spread blankets on the roadside and pulled her from the car. I squirted the gel. All of it. Every tube that I had. I dosed with the emergency, last resort, Glucagon shot. Teddy cried and howled in his crate in the car. I held and fanned my daughter, protecting her body with mine. Gradually, the seizure resolved and we continued on.

When we finally made it to the Oklahoma-Texas state line, four families from the previous experience greeted us. Those of us who had survived the unnatural disaster in Missouri had obvious signs of post-traumatic stress. It was a difficult time: not only were we back in the classroom with unproven, untrained dogs, but we had no idea what we were doing, or if training a diabetic alert dog was even possible. It was all a great big behavioral science experiment.

Our trainers taught us the basics of breaking down complex commands into bite-sized pieces. We started with the rudiments like "sit," "place," and "potty." We round-tabled and brainstormed to come up with ideas for how exactly to scent-train a DAD. One child's eyes always streamed when she experienced a low. The tears were caught on cotton squares. Another child salivated profusely; that, too, was captured. Ciara got sweaty feet, so we did clean cotton socks placed on her during a low. We tried different containers to protect the scent—glass saltshakers—for example. We threw all the ideas that we had gathered from talking to the experts on the table, weeded through them, and came up with game plans. Each dog was an experiment. Each dog was a glimmer of hope. None of us felt the conviction of imminent success: this was a venture into the wilds.

Just a few days into training, I went to take a shower. As I came back into the bedroom, I saw tiny four-month-old Teddy Bear sitting on Ciara's chest. Her test kit was in his mouth and he was wagging his tail exuberantly. I took the kit from him and checked Ciara's blood. The meter read 70. "Good low, Teddy Bear!" And I sobbed. I sobbed incredulity; I sobbed thanksgiving. Teddy Bear's pores exuded pride and joy as he received his well-deserved "Good Boy!" as if it were a medal of honor. Ciara woke with a smile to our odd celebration—my red, tear-streaked face, Teddy Bear's glowing, good-boy smile.

Ciara had loved Bo with all of the expectations of a young teen's first encounter with requited love. So now, at a worldly-wise eight, she allowed Teddy Bear to cuddle up next to her, and she loved Teddy Bear in the guarded broken-hearted way that belongs to an older, more journeyed person.

It is hard to resist Teddy Bear, though. He is so sweet. His eyes are a warm brown that go from laughing to intense concern. He is an emotional and nuanced pup, and he expresses his emotions through those chocolate eyes. When his eyes aren't enough, he whole-body wags his joy, or he tries to form his lips into English sentences, so we will understand him.

The time I spend with him each morning out exercising is a wonderful meditation in all that is good and right in this world. I throw the ball, and Teddy bunches his muscles under him, racing across the yard, tongue dangling out the side of his mouth. Every cell in his body knows that this is why he exists: to gather, leap and fly. He loves for me to throw the ball into the bushes, where he retrieves it and then stands very still, except for a tail that laughs against the twigs and leaves, hiding from me like a toddler. He's thrilled when I call to him with the non-command, "Where's Teddy?" It's his candy.

The only thing he loves more than exercise is his bath. Every day after his ball game, I tell him, "Go take a bath, Teddy." He runs up the stairs and jumps into the tub, so that I can wash the sand and dirt from his paw pads. Once a week this turns into a full bath. He knows it's a full-bath day when I take off his collar. This is when I get in the tub with him and massage all of the kinks out of his muscles. The stress of his workweek washes down the drain with the suds. He gets to lie on my bed swaddled in towels, and sleeps deeply with his puppy dreams of chasing rabbits through the field and of meat-covered, special-occasion bones. It's his therapy time.

Teddy was never a destructive puppy, chewing the things in our house. He always tried to do right. When he got a bladder infection and could only make it as far as the door and no farther, he stood contritely next to the guilty puddle he had made. He was obviously embarrassed to do something we told him was bad. From the very beginning, Teddy was hungry for affection and worked hard to figure out how to make us happy.

Teddy Bear's desire to please was coupled with forceful intelligence. I have come to rely on this. I've never pretended to be a trainer or have any inkling as to what to do. Training a DAD was more complicated than I had imagined when we were in the hospital. I had imagined that it was a matter of having an obedient dog that was trained in scent work and had a given method for alerting its handler. Our group discovered that DAD work is not at all straightforward. Our dogs had to be comfortable going anywhere that our children went. They had to have model obedience, but they also had to be disobedient. Here's a problem: when a diabetic starts to go low, their brains don't function in the normal way. The alert dog must be persistent and not give up the alert. If a diabetic with a low says, "Stop! Lie down!" the alert dog has to disregard this order and continue the alert or go find someone to help. The dog must be able to figure out when to obey and when to disobey. How do you teach situational disobedience?

Here's another problem: Statistics show that one third of the population in the United States has diabetes. In any given situation, our dog smells low BG numbers and high BG numbers and our dog can only focus on and alert the BG numbers that belong to his child. How do you train a hound to ignore all of the rabbits in a forest and only chase the little brown one that is his rabbit to watch?

Then there are the scents. We couldn't just train Teddy to alert to an 80. We needed to know if the number was anything along the number line below our given mark. Teddy, by the way, decided that he did not like Ciara to go below 100 and that is his mark now. We had trained him to 80, but Teddy is a strong-minded dog with his own thoughts on the subject. Throughout training, Teddy gave his input and since his ideas were usually far superior to mine, we welcomed his collaboration. Teddy felt that Ciara was safer with an alert at 100, so 100 it became.

To teach Teddy to alert to particular numbers, we played a game that I called "the perfect scent." It became his absolute favorite. When I was testing Ciara's blood, if the number ever came up 180, the perfect number for a high alert, or 100 for a low alert, I would lay Ciara on the ground and hide treats all over her. In her hair. In her clothes. Under her back. Teddy would clamber all over her sniffing, snuffing, snorting to find every single treat. The whole time I praised him with a happy, high-pitched voice. Very soon, Teddy would start dancing around Ciara when she was at those numbers. He was understanding the scent.

One day Ciara was outside with Teddy and her numbers dropped rapidly. I heard screaming in the back yard and ran with the test kit. There was tiny Teddy Bear, locked onto Ciara's sleeve, dragging her towards the house and help. I checked Ciara's blood and sure enough, she needed juice. Now! Teddy was whole-body wagging his victory and Ciara was sobbing, with long scratches down her arm where Teddy's teeth had reached for a hold of fabric. We needed a good alert.

***

Picking an alert is problematic. Each team in our group of seat-of-the pants, trying-to figure-this-out Midwest refugees worked on developing the right vocabulary. After the outside drag-you-to safety jumble, I decided on a bark. A loud bark when we were outside. A silent bark when we were inside. But barking as a signal was a no-go. In the first place Teddy loves to bark at the squirrels and other scampering wild things in our yard. I could never tell if Ciara was in trouble or if Teddy was in pursuit. Then there was the day when Teddy (correctly) alerted a low in the car with a sudden high-pitched bark right beside my ear that had me pulling off the road into a ditch. I had to find a different signal.

Our group was experimenting with bringsels, the little oblong stuffed pillows that our dogs could get and bring to us. When we saw bringsels in their mouths, it was time to check blood. When I made and presented these to Teddy, he almost sighed in relief. "Thank goodness," his body said. There was no training period. He got it with the first demonstration. This, he could do. He loved the bringsels. He loved to put as many as he could fit into his mouth and bring them all to me. They stuck out of his muzzle like fat neon-orange cigars, seven, eight, nine at a time. Teddy soon decided that he should stuff the bringsels into a shoe and present the shoe full of bringsels as his alert. This was helpful, because Teddy could drop the shoe and get our attention even if we were distracted. I think the whole shoe bit came from Teddy training on socks. He associated bringing foot smells to us with receiving his paycheck, a salmon-flavored cat treat.

Teddy has also learned that if a bringsel can't be found, socks and shoes work just as well. Better even. My husband is hard to distract from his task-at-hand. I have heard the shoe drop and drop and drop and have gone upstairs to find out why no one was heeding the alert, to see Teddy jump up on the bed and thump Todd in the head with the shoe. Teddy will get the job done.

Teddy also figured out that the bringsel alert is not always effective. He can't use it in the car, and he can't use it when he is under my feet. So he devised alternatives. If I am sitting down, Teddy will tap my foot with his. The more urgent the BG issue, the more intense the patting. Sometimes if Ciara is purposefully high for dance or Tae Kwon Do, Teddy will drape a knowing foot over mine. He wants me to know she is high, but he understands that we are not going to do anything about it. When she goes under the 180 mark, he will pull his foot back and curl into a ball to relax. When we are in the car, he will scratch at the plastic on the door, so I can hear that there is an issue.

It's when we're walking that Teddy has the most trouble. When we are in stores and all of those people with all of those yummy smells clinging to them walk by, Teddy has to focus very hard on his good behavior. His nose will sometimes lead his head over to the particular glory of a dog lover's pant-leg. He has to put a lot of effort into self-control in the dog-food section. It is often not until we stop and are still that Teddy can get the alert to go along with the good behavior. I have learned to stop frequently and give him the opportunity to shift his focus.

Teddy proved to be an overachiever. He made it his business

to keep Ciara on the narrow path of safety. He soon learned our military-regimen eating routine. He would come to get me if we were missing our designated meal. It's even hard for me to keep track of all that. Sadly, poor Teddy doesn't have a reset button, so twice a year he has a few days of confusion when daylight savings time has us springing forward or falling back.

Teddy has learned to listen for beeps. He knows not to stop alerting until the meter beeps out a reading. He knows to wait patiently for his "Good boy!" and his cat treat. He knows he must wait twenty minutes before he alerts again that a low he alerted to wasn't fixed. He knows that if the number is high, and he hears the beep for the check and another beep for insulin going in, then he must wait for an hour before he can alert us that the insulin dose was insufficient. His internal clock is rarely off.

At some point Teddy's training and learning seemed to go beyond what I can rationally understand. It seems to go to an ancient pack-mentality, and he can do things that could only be described as psychic. On a trip to Epcot, Teddy alerted when Ciara was 140. She should have been fine, but Teddy's posture, and the look in his eye, left nothing to doubt something awful was about to happen. I opened juice after juice until there were no more; I handed Ciara box of candy after box of candy until she cried with a tummy ache, and Teddy finally lay down next to me, exhausted. I calculated that I gave Ciara ninety carbs; that is two meals' worth of carbohydrates and her BG read 82. Can you imagine what would have happened if Teddy hadn't known how much food it would take to keep Ciara safe?

The very next day at Disney, Ciara wanted to go on the indoor roller coaster. I did not. A roller coaster was too much of a metaphor for my life to make it fun for me. We checked Ciara's blood; she was a very safe 150. Off she went with her dad. Meanwhile, I took Teddy to go potty. Mid-stream, Teddy stopped and went still with concentration. Suddenly, he took off running so fast that I was at the end of his lead hanging on.

He pulled me along, passed the place where Ciara had entered, down the block, around another building, through the hedges and there he stopped. I was perplexed; where were we? About thirty seconds later, Ciara and her dad came out through a side door of the building, right where we were standing. Teddy jumped up to my face and yipped. I had never seen this before. I checked Ciara's blood; she had dropped over a hundred points, down to 47, in nine minutes. She was on the verge of a seizure. Teddy saved the day. Again. He is our every-single-day hero.

For Teddy, Disney was sometimes a difficult experience, bringing so many curious hands that desperately wanted to pat his head. When we are out and about, Teddy always gets lots of attention. Usually it's positive, people just wanting to understand. We got some strange questions: "What's wrong with your daughter? She looks normal," and "Help that woman to her car; can't you see she's blind?" Sometimes the attention we got was unwelcome. A male security guard chased me into the ladies' room once and banged on my stall door, telling me to get my dog out of the restroom. My reply belied the "ladies" sign on the door. Once, the police were called on us. I was appreciative when they came, because I knew that we had the law on our side. The policemen weren't so sure. They thought it was probably reasonable that we leave the dog in the car while we were at the Baskin Robbins. It takes a lot of patience to deal with the public. It's not a lot of fun.

Being with a service dog is a lot like parenting a toddler—without the temper tantrums. Of course, the better the dog's training, the easier this task becomes. As awesome as Teddy is, I sadly made many mistakes training him when he was a baby. These mistakes are now part of his repertoire of behaviors. Some of these bad habits are dangerous. For example, when he was a puppy and we were on asphalt, I would run with him into the grass to get him excited about going potty before we went into a store. Now when I say "potty" and we're on the macadam, Teddy takes off running, as he had been trained to do. He's a seventy-five pound dog racing for the patch of grass. I can't let Ciara walk him; it's too dangerous.

Some of those early bad training habits are funny. One of the first alerts I tried to teach Teddy, with absolutely no foresight, was to circle through my legs to get my attention. It wasn't a great alert, and the bringsel and foot tapping quickly took its place—except when Teddy becomes very excited about a low. To this day, when Teddy has an exciting "low hit," he will try to dance through my legs in private or public, in pants or a skirt. Our big old Teddy Bear circles through my legs like a puppy, much to everyone's glee and my embarrassment.

One of the things that I never was able to teach Teddy was how to walk on a lead outside of a store. In the store, Teddy was an angel. Outside of the store, Teddy wanted to be the alpha, take the lead, and pull me through life. This became difficult the bigger and stronger he became. Then came a series of unfortunate events. It started with an English boxer as tall as the six-year-old walking him, a boxer who had been trained to protect the family's children from other dogs. He stood sentry on the soccer field path. When we rounded the corner, he sprang on Teddy's back. Even as I choked the boxer into submission, he was able to rip off the medical bags that Teddy carried. Teddy and I were both shaking when we got in the car. That was a Tuesday.

That Saturday I took my Girl Scout troop on a hike in the state park. As I turned to count heads, I saw a flash of white fur sail past and land on Teddy's back. I used my backpack to sledgehammer the massive dog. The straps on my backpack gave out before the dog did. The other moms all put hands in the fight and pulled the dog off Teddy, who lost another backpack to the onslaught and had a rip near his tail. Teddy now saw other dogs as the enemy. He couldn't be near them without raising his hackles and baring his teeth with a warning growl.

The next week, Ciara, Teddy, and I went to pick up a pizza. A teen in his jacked-up car screeched into the parking spot next to where I stood with Teddy at my side, as I juggled cardboard boxes in one hand and my keys in the other. Teddy and I were both startled and frightened as we were sandwiched, unseen by the other driver, between his dually and my minivan. The teen ran in the store, leaving his engine thrumming loudly under the steady pound of the ear-drum-endangering subwoofer. His whole truck vibrated against us. I was able to get the back door to slide open. Teddy hurled himself inside. I crawled in after him, over the console, unable to open my door wide enough to get in.

Before all of this, Teddy had been difficult on the lead; now he was impossible. His head swung left and right. He crouch-ran in preparation for the next scary, horrible thing to land on him. He dragged me through parking lots and parks. It was an impossible situation. I called everyone I could think of. I read every article I could find. Most people said that this many traumas in such a short period were probably not reversible. One man said different: Mike Stewart.

***

In a tear-stained conversation with Rachel Thornton, a member of the make-it-all-better band of moms, I related our distress and that I believed it was cruel to take Teddy out in public; and, it was physically too much for me. Rachel suggested that she talk to the Wildrose folks. The Wildrose staff had been helping Rachel and her daughter, Abi, train Teddy's brother, Mr Darcy. Imagine their luck to live only a little more than an hour's drive away from Mike Stewart, one of the world's foremost hunting dog trainers. Imagine our luck that Mike has a hugely caring and generous heart. Rachel called me back with an invitation to go down to Mississippi for help.

It was January 2010 and Teddy was nearly two years old. We had been on many adventures together; this was the make-or-break one for our diabetic alert team. As soon as the invitation came, I was throwing clothes into suitcases and kissing my husband goodbye. With two kids and Teddy Bear, I aimed my minivan back over the mountains and across the states for the two-day drive. We arrived to bitterly cold weather. Ice-sparkled air wavered between the low teens and the single digits the week we worked at Wildrose. I barely felt it, being so concentrated on the task at hand.

Mike Stewart first assessed me walking Teddy, who was as bad as he could be. Teddy paid zero attention to me, as he snuffled the delicious scents of the dogs, ducks, and deer, which had recently passed by. Teddy nearly dumped me into the ice-covered pond. Mike chuckled under his breath. "Well, there isn't anything wrong with this dog," he said.

"It's you." Mike took me inside and started laying out the fundamentals of just how I was ruining Teddy Bear.

The first problem started when he was a baby and all of the trainers had told me how important it was for Teddy to have "downtime" and "time off." So sometimes he was treated like a service dog and sometimes he was treated like a pet. When we went out to play, I let Teddy Bear set the pace and tell me what he wanted to do. So sometimes I was the dominant alpha dog and sometimes Teddy was. These conflicting messages confused Teddy. When he was attacked by other dogs Teddy hadn't been clear about where he was in the pecking order and what his role should be. He wasn't confident that I would protect him. The anxiety of these conflicting messages along with the burden of being perfectly behaved most times and intelligently misbehaving at other times was too stressful for Teddy Bear.

Mike had me fill out a chart with a schedule of a normal day. In one column, I wrote out our behaviors; in the other, what behaviors I wanted to see. It was right there in black and white how I was confusing Teddy Bear. Mike laid the tasks in front of me.

When Teddy was on the leash, Mike used a martingale lead and no tagged collar. At first I balked, but Mike pointed out that all of the other leads I had used had left Teddy blistered and choked. Mike also pointed out that in a pack there was a natural consequence for misbehavior; this was just a replication.

To my surprise, it only took a correction or two and Teddy was walking steadily next to Mike. Very soon after that, Mike had Teddy walking off lead with a dually pickup truck heading up the driveway at them. I cringed as I watched for Teddy's reaction. Teddy understood that Mike was in charge and Mike would keep him safe. Mike was right; Teddy was fine. It was all me.

Teddy and I practiced walking. A lot. We also practiced playing. If I were to be in charge of Teddy's wellbeing, then Teddy was never to be in charge of me. This was true except for that particular disobedience I needed from him when it came to blood sugar numbers. When Teddy is on the scent, Teddy is in charge.

Quickly, Teddy learned that alerting is the only time he is allowed to push his agenda. Everywhere else, I'm head of the pack. Instead of my mindlessly throwing the ball for Teddy, we now have a series of ball games that we play. Teddy sits and waits for a command, and he is rewarded with a ball toss. Don't get me wrong; this is still a joyous time for both of us, with Teddy running in the pure bliss of the chase. Now he knows that if I yell "candy," that he's performed a task really well, and he gets to go into the bushes and wiggle his tail as he hides. But I am in charge of the games. When I call "last one, Teddy," Teddy brings the ball back to the door where he puts it away and waits for his next happy command, "Teddy, go take a bath."

Mike asked me to stop petting Teddy so much, because indiscriminant affection can dilute the reward system. This is one that I don't follow as well as I should. Petting Teddy is like medication to me when I'm stressed. Mike also asked us to stop giving Teddy his cat treats, and I understood the thought process. In Teddy's world, for almost two years, there had been a rhythm to the alerts. For almost two years, Teddy had been rewarded with treats for his alerts. Taking the treat out put a "What did I do wrong?" light into Teddy's chocolate brown eyes. I just couldn't stop giving him treats for alerts.

For a week Mike, Teddy, and I tried to work out all of the kinks that had coiled themselves into Teddy's temperament. A harder task was for Mike to get me to step away from my soft, seat-of-the pants, amorphous personality. When we left Wildrose, Teddy was a much more stable dog, one that could walk confidently in a parking lot with cars buzzing by or walk carefully through a museum. He could hike the woods without a shiver or a shake, and he could stand a few tentative get-to-know you sniffs from other dogs.

✳✳✳

Of all the places Teddy goes, his favorite is to go with Ciara to dance class. All the girls know not to touch him when he's in his service vest. Teddy scootches his bottom to the very edge of his blanket and reaches his muzzle towards them, hoping they will get close enough that he can give them a surreptitious and affectionate lick on the hand. And when they have all come to say hi and tell him how wonderful he is, Teddy settles back on his place to watch Ciara, and pat, pat, pat my foot as an alert when I need to pull her off the floor with a soft whistle.

Though Teddy Bear is definitely Ciara's dog, I am his main handler. Ciara will take over when she is out and about without me—but that is rare. Handling Teddy is a huge responsibility. At age eleven, Ciara was not focused enough to take on this duty. There were constant issues with public access and the public's behavior. There is the required attention to Teddy's conduct and safety. There is also the attention that needs to be paid to the alert and the follow-up. Even with me there saying, "Alert Ciara, check your blood," it takes some pestering on my part. When you're chatting with your friends, or dancing your heart out, it's hard to stop and listen to your mom or your dog. It's hard to want to prick your finger and check for the twentieth time that day. It's tedious to do the math for an insulin dose if you're high, to eat when you're not hungry, or drink juice when you're not thirsty. By spring 2010, we were doing great. The kids and I were heading back down to Mississippi to help the Wildrose crew with a DAD training weekend and I was very excited to show off our progress to Mike. Ciara, my son, Aiden, Teddy, and I were planning to travel around the United States for the next six weeks. Wildrose was just our first stop. We planned to head out on Thursday.

On Monday of that week, I heard Teddy Bear cooing to me to come check Ciara's blood. It was three in the morning. I checked, "Good low, Teddy." But Teddy's head was doing something strange. I could see him shaking it back and forth in the dark. When I gave him his treat, the shaking stopped. I went back to bed, and Teddy called me again. I checked, gave another juice, and turned to see Teddy looking at me with lost eyes, having a seizure. I had my husband load Teddy into my minivan, as I got hurriedly dressed. Once again, I was driving for help. All of the memories of driving Ciara to the hospital in her coma flooded through me. All of the fear that I could not keep her safe pinged like subatomic particles, ricocheting around my brain. When I pulled up to the animal emergency hospital, Teddy seemed fine. I explained what had happened. The vet ran tests. He couldn't find anything wrong. Then Teddy had another seizure. This time it didn't stop, and they had to medicate Teddy with Valium.

In the exam room, that first night of Teddy's seizures, I was once again almost hysterical with grief. I was remembering vividly Ciara's seizures. The hospital smells transported me back to that night when I ran—hobbled behind my comatose daughter. The cold green tiles that had danced to my left and right on that long run behind the gurney were the same institutional green tiles that I was leaned against with doped-up Teddy lying awkwardly in my lap. I felt the same desperation as I hugged Teddy, anchoring him to this world with the weight of my need for everything to be all right. For him to be all right. He was Ciara's safety. He was our respite, our healing balm; we needed him. I thought about the irony and the full circle I had traveled.

Since the emergency vet didn't know how to help us, I was referred to a neurologist in Washington, D.C. Teddy was seizing with more frequency. It plucked at every nerve as I drove to D.C., trying to maintain my focus, trying to exude strength and confidence for all of us. The doctors spent long hours observing Teddy, just as the doctors had spent long hours observing Ciara. I made sure that they checked Teddy for diabetes.

As we sat, watched, and waited, I told the doctors our Teddy's stories of heroism. After observing several seizures, they did an MRI and a spinal tap. Thank goodness for good insurance! Even drunkenly walking into the waiting room after the procedures, Teddy came over to get a bringsel and alert. "Take that one with a grain of salt, ma'am. Your dog is flying pretty high on his meds," the doctor said. I knew better; I knew Teddy alerted from a place untouchable by the medications. Sure enough, Ciara was 67. "Good low, Teddy! Treat!"

They found that Teddy was systemically healthy. They weren't sure what was going on with him or why this was happening. I groaned. Again? This was playing out just like Ciara's nightmare. The doctors counseled me that it was in Teddy's best interest to continue with our plans to travel. The doctors felt that challenging Teddy's brain to adapt, and adapt some more, was the best therapy for him.

Teddy Bear had his last seizure the night before we got to

Wildrose. There never was a rhyme or reason. We got to help with the new DAD puppies. I was thrilled that all of these families, through Wildrose's efforts, were now going to feel the same relief I feel having Teddy walking vigilantly by Ciara's side. At the end of the weekend, we packed the tents, loaded up the minivan, and headed west. A lifestyle made possible by the sweet intellect of our beloved Teddy Bear. All these years later, we are still adventuring. Teddy is still whole-body wagging when he hears his "Good boy!" And Ciara is still seizure-free. An answer to my prayers.

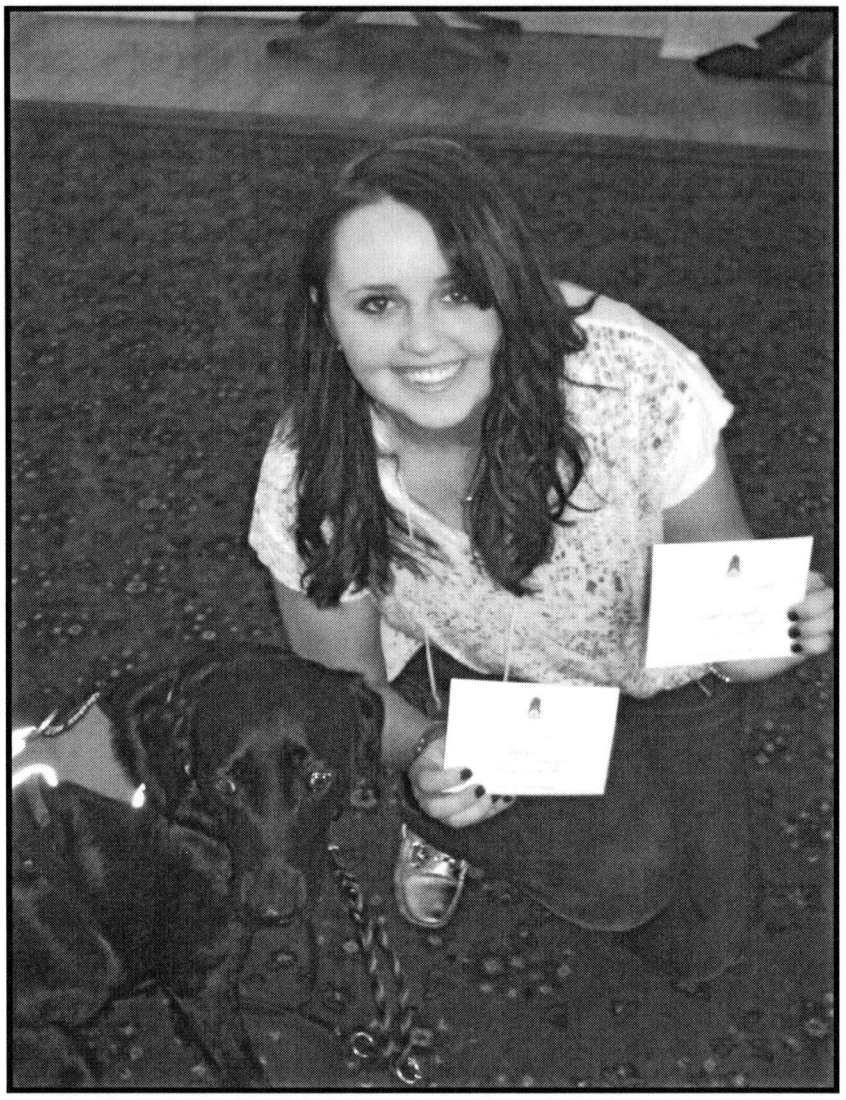

Olive with Devon Wright.

Olive and Devon Wright: Team Empathy

MY LIFE BECAME COMPLICATED WHEN I was twelve. I remember my mom walking through the door of Ms. Pavlik's seventh grade humanities classes. My mom told me to grab my bag and we quickly walked to our green Volvo. When we sat down in the car, my Mom gave me nine or ten assorted sheets of medical papers and I glanced down at them as I got buckled up. Before my Mom put the car in drive she took a deep breath and said, "Devon, you've been diagnosed with diabetes." The first thing that came to my head was, *No, I can't be sick, people like me just don't get sick.* I was a healthy twelve-year-old. I rode horses, I danced, and I had numerous friends and a great family. I was *not* sick.

My mom and I sat in silence for the twenty-minute drive to the hospital. The nurse led us to an examining room and stuck a sharp needle into my thumb. As she squeezed my thumb, a droplet of blood bubbled on the tip. When she left, I examined my thumb for damage. A small scab had formed on the tip and I showed my teary-eyed mother my wound. Those "wounds" would become a daily occurrence. From there we went to the emergency room to start an IV.

***

Looking back on this day, I realize how sick I had really been. I was wetting the bed. I was constantly dehydrated and no amount of water could satisfy my thirst. I was constantly hungry, but too nauseous to eat. From the moment I was diagnosed, nothing would be the same. I would struggle with testing, injections, and taking care of myself every day for the rest of my life.

When I turned thirteen, I started on an insulin pump, a medical device attached to my body that constantly administers insulin. My A1C, the average amount of sugar in my cells over the last ninety days, was at an all-time best. However, despite having excellent control of my diabetes, I was suffering emotionally. As everyone who attended middle school knows, middle school girls can be mean and my diabetes was the butt of numerous jokes and pranks. With my pump, I believed that everyone could see the disease I had and know that I was sick. I was not comfortable feeling so transparent. Even though I had three close friends at my small school, most of the girls in my class were hurtful and mean. Most of the kids in my class believed that diabetes was contagious and some even refused to talk to me. In eighth grade someone put a death threat in my cubby. I don't think at the time the girls in my class or I understood the gravity of the note, but I did understand that people disliked me because of something I couldn't control. I was in emotional turmoil and I saw a child counselor to help me think through my feelings.

I decided to transfer from the school I had attended through eighth grade. In high school, people were much more understanding and did not make fun of my diabetes, but I still felt self-conscious wearing an insulin pump. I stayed on the pump until my sophomore year of high school when I decided to switch back to injections.

After I ditched the pump, my blood sugars were terrible,

but nobody knew I was diabetic. During my senior year of high school I tightened up my control by testing more and becoming more regular on giving shots.

Riding has always been my passion and I love spending time with horses. Throughout much of my childhood and teenage years, I competed on a national level in equestrian. I ride English and execute jumps. In my sophomore year of high school I began working with a trainer in Parker, Colorado, two-and-a-half hours east of Vail and just south of Denver. During weekends I commuted, and in the summers I lived in Parker with my trainer, competing all across Colorado, as well as Arizona, California, and some of the East Coast. Baylor University recruited me to ride on their NCAA D1 equestrian team. So I decided to attend Baylor in Waco, Texas.

I enjoyed the college equestrian team, but it also put stress on me that I had never experienced before, both mental and physical. Not only was I doing more physical activity, I was also working hard as a college student at a difficult school. This had a negative impact on my diabetes. The workouts gave me severe post-workout lows and the stress from the team drama as well as academics produced bad adrenalin and consequently dangerously high blood sugars.

As you can imagine, my freshman year at college was difficult. At home I had relied a great deal on my parents, close friends, and equestrian coach to help manage my diabetes. They could tell when I was high or low because of my behavior. When I went to Baylor, I knew a few people but no one that I was close to. Twice during my first year I passed out from low blood sugar. Because I developed hypoglycemic unawareness, I could not tell when I was dropping. One time in the middle of the night my hypoglycemia was so severe that we had to call an ambulance to my dorm because I suddenly collapsed to the floor. My roommates knew that I was diabetic, but they didn't know emergency protocol. Luckily, they called my parents and tested my blood sugar and discovered that I was at a dangerously low level. They then called an ambulance. That episode was a wake-up call. My situation obviously put unnecessary stress on my parents, my roommates, my coaches, and me. I was afraid to go low and I became obsessive about not dropping, fearful that I could easily drop into a dangerous zone without even knowing. Veteran diabetics know it is unrealistic for diabetics to not go low.

I stopped giving myself the correct dosage of insulin so that I could stay at a higher level. This is dangerous for both short-term and long-term health. Being at an elevated level made it difficult for me to compete on the equestrian team as well as focus on my academics. When you are high, you experience symptoms like fatigue, extreme thirst, lack of hunger, and frequent urination. Moreover, it is incredibly hard to concentrate on anything when you are high; it is like a blockade. You want to focus, but something is holding you back. Even though you can read and understand the words, it doesn't "click." Being a driven person, I am passionate about doing well, sometimes to the point of harming myself more than helping. This was the case with my obsession over low blood sugars. I was creating a new problem, and it was flowing over into other aspects of my life.

***

Before I went to college, my parents and I had talked briefly about getting a diabetic alert dog, a DAD. I decided that I didn't want one at college because it would be extra work and because I was still self-conscious about having diabetes. However, halfway through my freshman year, my erratic sugars convinced me I didn't want to live my life in fear of a chronic disease, so we did some research about DADs.

My dad's friend, Andy, had a gundog named Wildrose Rio, who was trained at Wildrose Kennels in Mississippi. At the Teva Mountain Games held annually in Vail, my dad and Andy ran into Wildrose's president Mike Stewart and they talked about DADs. My dad enthusiastically came home to get me so I could meet Mike. However by the time we got back to the games, Mike had left.

In the following days over dinner, we discussed how having a dog could help me out. I liked the idea of the dog, but I didn't like the idea of the attention a service dog would attract. Later on, when I decided that I was interested in a diabetic alert dog, my parents and I gathered information from the Wildrose website and spoke to Rachel Thornton from Wildrose about getting a DAD. In early November I submitted my application for a DAD, which consisted of pages of questions as well as blood sugar logs and a week's worth of activities.

Rachel interviewed me by phone, because I was in Texas at school. I was nervous, because this was a really big deal. It was like a job interview, but for something that could change my quality of life. Rachel reached me on my cell phone when I was walking back from class to my dorm. As I talked with her, I paced back and forth across the huge grass quadrangle called Fountain Mall on Baylor's campus. When the interview was over, I had no idea how it went. Rachel told me they were hesitant to give DADs to college students because they are so busy and most don't have time for that type of responsibility. However, I had also made it clear that I was not interested in partying and that I was very driven and focused on academics and the equestrian team. Rachel and I kept in close contact for the next few months, and in early May, after I finished my freshman year, my mom and I decided to visit Wildrose in Mississippi for a DAD workshop. We went unmatched with a dog just to see if this was something I was interested in. I was still skeptical about it until we got there.

After my last final exam, my mom and I flew to Jackson, Mississippi, and then drove to the DAD conference in Oxford. Arriving a couple of minutes late, we sat down at a table in the front of the room, where Rachel was giving an introduction to the weekend. There were about thirty people sitting in the room, with their DADs lying quietly on the floor while Rachel talked. As we took our seats, I looked around at all the dogs that could save lives. There was a sweet yellow Lab sitting in front of us on a mat. After I had been there for about fifteen minutes, Charlie grabbed a bringsel that was attached to his leash. All the people nearby pulled out their meters to test. It turned out that *I* was the one he was alerting! When a dog alerts you, it is magical. My skepticism disappeared after his alert. It was eye opening for me to discover first-hand that another animal can tell me something that my body doesn't even know.

During the workshop there was a lot of lecturing about things that I didn't really understand at the time. However, I also worked with Mike and Rachel Thorton, doing activities with dogs that I borrowed. Rachel and Mike must have seen something in me, because on the last day Rachel asked if I'd like to take a dog with me for the summer. I was surprised, but I think that Rachel and Mike saw that I was comfortable with the dogs because of my background with horses.

We decided that Olive was the best match for me, and she came to me on June 10. Olive is the sister to Deke, Mike's personal dog and the Ducks Unlimited mascot. Rachel flew out to Colorado for twenty-four hours to drop Olive off and give me some tips and information about living with a DAD. I was so excited walking through the airport to pick up Rachel and Oli. We rode the elevator down to my car and Rachel talked about how "soft" Olive is and how important it is to acclimate her into my world slowly. Together, we visited places where I typically spend time. At the stable where I ride we went out to the barn to make sure Olive would be okay around horses, and then we drove up the mountains to my home. Rachel spent the night observing Olive and me, making sure that we were a good match.

All summer Olive and I worked diligently as a team, focusing on her confidence during alerting. Olive had wonderful obedience skills because of her hunting training background. However, because her initial training limited her "retrieving" only on verbal command, Olive was not very confident in grabbing the bringsel to alert. This was never a problem for me with her, though, because I have always been able to read her subtle hints as to when my blood sugar is off. Her cues were not initially consistent, but because I spend close to every minute with her, those subtle hints become alarm bells. From the very beginning Olive and I communicated well. I always understood when she was alerting: she would sit up abruptly from being down, or gently nudge my leg a few times in a row. It is difficult to articulate the exact things she does when she alerts because it is like a conversation with us. She is always attentive, but if I am a little high or low, she will be intently interested in what I am doing. It is as if we share the same brain. Some people can't even tell that she is alerting, but I can because of the way that she focuses on me, and stops caring about anything else.

During the summer trial period Rachel and I kept in touch daily via text, email, or phone calls. I sent her a weekly log of my sugar levels and Olive's alerts. At the end of July I was supposed to send Olive back to Wildrose. It was a somber day. My dad drove my mom and me to meet Mike and Cathy at the Vail Tivoli Lodge. I kept my composure in the car ride over, but when we were walking Olive to meet them, I was crying. Olive had really become one of the best things in my life and the thought of giving her back was heartbreaking. Olive and I have always been in touch emotionally, which is unique to our pair. My mom said that when we were walking to Mike and Cathy, both Oli and I looked disheartened.

As we reached Mike and Cathy, I tried to pull myself together. We spent about an hour talking about dogs and Olive and how great she was. My mood lightened a little bit and Olive's followed. She actually alerted me then, which I noticed, even though nobody else did. Mike had been watching us and commented on the subtlety of our communication. As we neared the end of our time together, Mike told me that they didn't really have a place for Olive at the kennels just then and that it would help them out if I could keep her until October when some space opened up. I had mixed feelings about this. I was ecstatic because I wouldn't have to say goodbye to Olive yet, but I was also wary, because eventually I would still have to say goodbye to my doe-eyed black Lab.

***

Back home Olive and I carried on as usual with my activities, including horse training. About a week after meeting with the Stewarts, I received a wonderful email from Rachel saying that I could keep Olive as my DAD if I chose. I remember reading the email on my iPhone after a long day at a horse show and bursting into tears. It came as a complete surprise. I should have guessed something was up when Mike had driven an hour and a half to tell me that I could keep the dog for another few months. The day I found out I would be Oli's forever home is one of my favorite moments with her and something I truly cherish. Olive kept me safe all summer and gave me a confidence I had struggled to find before. I was no longer afraid to give shots, or go low because I knew that I had a little furry angel looking out for me at all times.

We signed the paperwork with the Stewarts and I contacted the university as well as the owner of the apartment complex where I would be living my sophomore year. Baylor asked for proof that she is a service dog, so I registered her and we went off to college, ready to begin my second year. I also emailed all of my professors, letting them know I that I would have a service animal and that she would not be a distraction in their classrooms.

Having a service dog did not stigmatize me after all, but

actually helped me meet people. Olive went everywhere with me and became a celebrity on campus. My teachers and classmates alike loved her sweet disposition. On a college campus, most people are educated enough to know not to pet Olive so I never had much of an issue with annoying questions that a handler receives frequently in public. Olive went to every class with me and sat at my feet or next to my desk. If I went to dinner and a movie, Olive went to dinner and the movie. She did incredibly well with college life, considering my inconsistent schedule. She was fine spending time at the library until the early hours of the morning; some days after staying up late she would even let me sleep in until nine. Olive attended football games and basketball games regularly with me. She brings so much joy to my life and it is fun to hear how she makes other people happy as well. Throughout the year I posted pictures and stories about our life together on my Facebook page.

All of us who take DADs out in the public experience random incidents. Last fall I was grocery shopping in Target and a little boy came running up to me and tapped me on the leg. I am used to refusing adorable toddlers and young children and I thought he was going to ask to pet Olive. I turned to him and crouched down a little bit and he whispered to me, "I know your dog is only wearing that vest because it's a Power Ranger... but don't worry, I won't tell anyone." I winked at him and he ran away giggling. Small encounters like that always brighten my day.

At college Olive and I continued to thrive in many aspects, but we also struggled with stress and too little time separated. Separation is an important element of a relationship, too. In early September I was admitted into the ICU because of a stomach bug, which had quickly developed into DKA (diabetic ketoacidosis), a complex condition involving high blood sugar level, overproduction of ketones, and high acid levels. Although I recovered, Olive was extremely anxious in the cramped hospital room during my stay. I was unable to communicate with her and hospital attendants were continuously coming and going, and working around me. In the days following my hospitalization, Olive remained disoriented. I tried to work through it with her, but being a college student requires lots of time and focus on schoolwork, and I continued to bring Olive into new situations, stressing her further. I spent loads of time and energy trying to "fix Olive up" by spending more time away from her, but also doing more fun things with her. However, Olive was either overzealous with her alerting and would alert when I wasn't really off, or she would stop alerting altogether.

I discussed my situation with Rachel, and we realized that Olive needed a break from me and some time away, where she could chill out and "reset." Eventually, I chose to send Olive back to Rachel for a while to take a "vacation." This was one of the hardest things Olive and I have had to face, but it was imperative for us as a team. I had to realize two things that every team must realize: first, our dogs are not robots, and they are allowed to make mistakes and to get stressed out; second, most teams do not consist of a DAD and a dog trainer. Because I have no knowledge of dog training except for the advice the Wildrose staff has given me, I cannot always fix problems.

Part of the reason Olive and I spiraled out of control so quickly is that we are extremely in-tune. I had no idea how much Olive fed off my energy until I met Rachel at the airport that year. I was obviously emotional when Olive was leaving, but I sat down with Rachel and talked for a while. Rachel observed that as I calmed, Olive followed. This was a reminder of how attentive Oli is to me. It is one of her strongest qualities, but it can also be a negative if she stresses because I do.

Rachel literally took Olive on a vacation. Olive traveled with other DADs on a family vacation to Washington, D.C. and Gettysburg, Pennsylvania. It proved to be a beneficial break for her, although I missed her so and was delighted when Wildrose's Mary Griffin brought her back to me and spent a couple of days observing our reunion. The time away from Olive reminded me that it is perfectly acceptable to ask for help. I learned that a handler needs to be able to be a strong person and help her dog by admitting she may not be able to fix everything herself. After Olive's vacation we began making some vital changes to our routine.

I scheduled more intentional separation from each other. Instead of fifteen minutes a day, it was more like two hours. Olive and I also began doing things together other than service dog work. We took an obedience class at PetSmart where we learned new tricks like "crawl," "bow," "shake," and "back up." This gave Olive and me something to do together that had nothing to do with diabetes. Olive and I also began working on Wildrose's Adventure Dog program, going kayaking, hiking, and horseback riding together. These activities give Olive something she can work at with me and receive attention from me, while taking a break from her job.

When Olive and I spent the Thanksgiving Holidays back at home in Vail, I had an opportunity to work with her during hunting season. My father was excited to take her out duck and pheasant hunting. My twin brothers Andrew and Michael and Dad's friend Andy, who owns Wildrose Rio, accompanied my father and me on our outing. The seven of us loaded into the car and drove a few hours into the Eastern Plains to hunt pheasants. Olive worked well as a retriever *and* a service dog that day.

When we arrived at the field to pheasant hunt, we threw a bumper with pheasant wings a couple times so that both Olive and Rio could pick up the scent. Then, we set out on the hunt in brisk mountain air with a bluebird sky overhead. Olive was outstanding and she was a joy to watch. She immediately went to work following Rio's lead, and together they flushed a number of roosters, which the shooters took. I quickly realized that when Olive retrieved her bird, it was very similar to when she alerts my low blood sugar. With her nose in the air, she was eagerly working in front of Dad and Andy. Once she caught the scent, she would flush the birds until a bird shot upwards into the sky.

During the hunt I began to get nervous about my blood sugar dropping because we were walking most of the day. My brother, Mike, had my blood meter and Skittles in his hunting vest. I started to notice that Olive became less interested in finding birds and more interested in what I was doing. She started walking closer to me and became very interested and anxious. At first I figured she was tired, and I blew her off. However, when she started disobeying direct commands and whining, I knew that I needed to test. The only problem was that at that point my brother, Mike, was on the other side of a swamp with my blood meter. There was no way either one of us could walk through it.

We tried having my brother call Olive in order to give her the Skittles and meter to bring back to me. However, because Olive was so concerned about me, she wouldn't leave my side. So we enlisted Rio to do the job. My brother called Rio over and put my blood meter in his mouth The Skittles were secured safely inside the waterproof casing. I called Rio back and he came bounding through the wet marsh with my blood meter. I tested my blood sugar and Olive was spot on about the low. My blood sugar was in the sixties and I quickly ate a few handfuls of Skittles.

This brings up an interesting question as to whether or not a diabetic alert dog is able to multitask. In Olive's case, the answer is a resounding "YES!" The fact that she stopped bounding around chasing after those delicious-smelling birds to alert me that was incredible. I am not sure that dogs have the ability to prioritize, but I do know that Olive is well aware of her service job and is a devoted and life-saving dog.

In the spring semester, during rush, Olive and I joined a sorority. Alpha Delta Pi welcomed us both with open arms and sorority life has been very exciting. Olive is the first dog in Baylor University Panhellenic history, as well as ADPi history, to ever participate in Greek life.

***

Having finished my sophomore year at college, Olive and I have returned home to Colorado for the summer. We attended summer school in Boulder, and hung out at home in Vail on the weekends. We have a pool in our backyard and for alert rewards and exercise Olive retrieves in the pool.

I was kidding around one afternoon saying that she could do Dock Dogs because she is such an excellent jumper. Then I looked online and figured out when the Dock Dog competition was in Vail. So she and I attended the Teva Mountain Games in Vail and competed in the Dock Dogs Big Air competition.

We got to the competition early in the morning so I could do a couple of practice runs with Olive. I wanted to know that she was comfortable jumping off the dock without any distractions before I asked her to do it with a lot of distractions. Olive was incredible. On the first throw she leapt off the dock and jumped in the water like a professional. Later that day we competed in the Big Air competition. Olive made it about eight-and-a-half feet, which, compared to some of the other dogs' jumps, was short. I was proud of her anyway. Her versatility and her confidence in me have really made leaps and bounds. Her poise in a variety of new life opportunities has increased during our time together, and she is a trustworthy companion. She has a special bond with me and will try anything I ask of her. We also attended Wildrose's Adventure Dog workshop that Mike conducted at Aspen. The AD workshop is an instructional event to practice all sorts of outdoor activities from trail hiking and biking to camping and kayaking. At the seminar, Olive practiced a number of skills we had already been working on, like kayaking, hiking, going to parties and networking. Olive also worked on some new skills, like running alongside a bike, camping, fishing, crossing rivers, and shed hunting—hunting for elk horns. We had a blast learning new skills as well as catching up with Mike and receiving a few reminders about the Wildrose Way. We got a great start on achieving merits for the AD certificate program.

Olive and I have continued to grow as a team and I cannot imagine life without her now. Not only has she changed my quality of life, but she has also changed my outlook. There is something about having an animal fighting for the same outcome with you. I have incredibly supportive family and friends, but Olive is with me all day. She knows the highs and lows of my life better than anyone else. My little black Labrador retriever keeps me safe and gives me comfort, and she also gives me hope.

Questions to Consider

For parents considering getting a DAD for a teen, here are some questions I encourage them to discuss with the teen before getting a service dog:

Are you and your teen willing to put the time and effort into working with a dog? Dogs are not machines and they are constantly changing. (I still spend a lot of time training Olive and making sure that she stays sharp.) Teens are busy and DADs are a lot of work.

Is your teen planning to have a big night life? It is not fair to drag your DAD to parties and bars into the wee hours of the morning. Animals need rest and cannot be expected to perform perfectly with minimum sleep, especially when a diabetic's blood sugars become erratic from drinking alcohol.

Is your child okay with receiving inordinate amounts of attention from strangers? People wonder about service dogs and they are going to come up and stare. It comes with the territory. You have a service dog and humans are naturally inquisitive. Also, people will come up and ask you questions. It gets old, but you have to be courteous and answer their questions. I get questions from many people every day.

All the pros of having a DAD far outweigh the cons. I am grateful that Wildrose is so dedicated to training these incredible animals. I can't imagine life without my guardian dog, and I am blessed to have an incredible support group for sweet Olive and me.

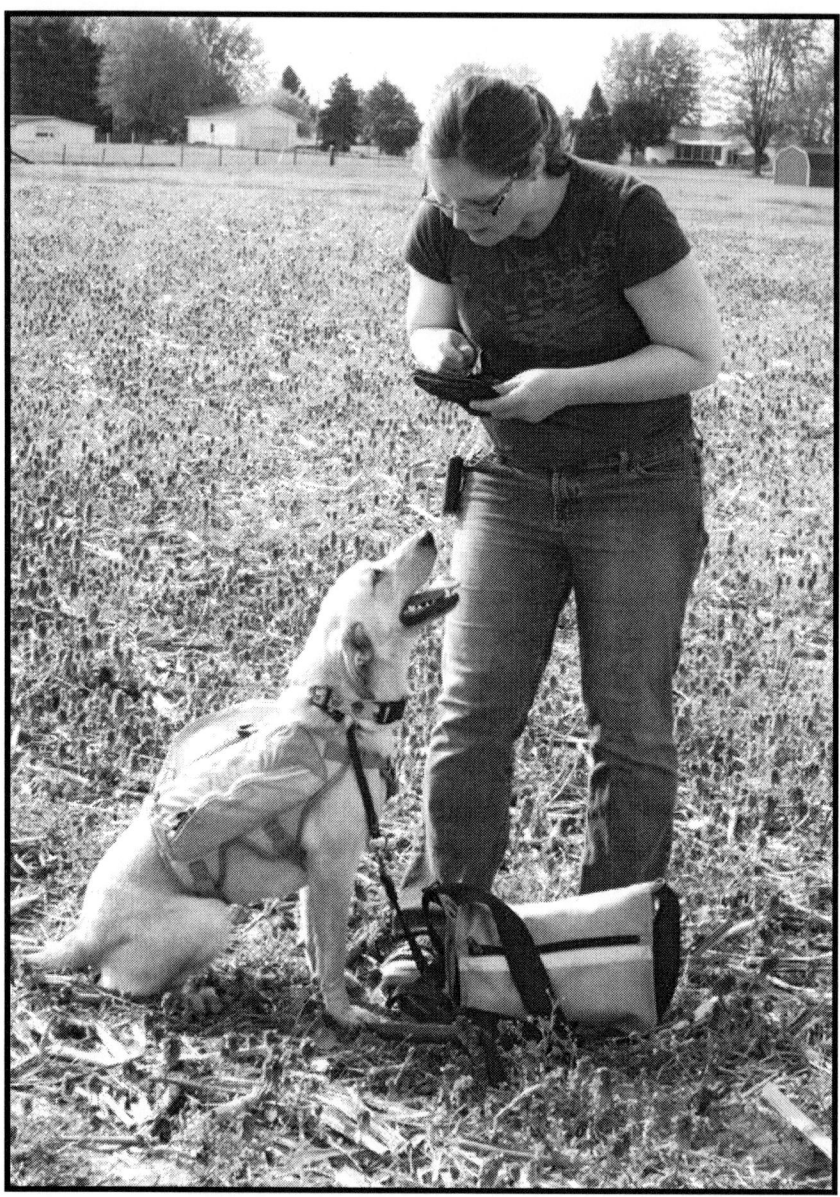

Juniper and Megan DeHaven.

Juniper and Megan DeHaven: Special Communication

MY LIFE CAREENED INTO UNCERTAINTY the week of Halloween that year. That week was beautiful as the rest of that fall had been: autumn in its full glory.

My mom and stepdad were out of town for a special occasion. My older sister, Allison, was left home to look after my older brother, Aaron, and me. I had been sick for a few days with something that seemed like the flu. In the moment between sleep and wakefulness I had a strange momentary flash of perception that there was something very wrong, immediately followed by agony. I began screaming in pain, not knowing what was going on. My sister was right there, trying to figure out what was wrong. It must have been startling for her to see me jump out of bed that way, doubled over, a crying, screaming mess. I was frantically moving around: standing, sitting, pacing. I was trying to understand what was happening, trying to make the pain stop. I would have done anything to stop it. My sister called my father and he came to get me. Sitting on the side of the bed, I was coping, trying to keep my mind together underneath the pain: ice picks in my kidneys, acid in my blood, sand in my mouth. I couldn't move. When my dad arrived and assessed the situation, he told me to get dressed, that we were going to the hospital. I told him that I couldn't... I couldn't move, couldn't get dressed, and couldn't walk. He had to pick me up and carry me out to the van. He drove to the closest hospital. By the time we arrived, I had mostly blacked out. I have some flashes of memory: lying in the back of the van, being carried into the hospital, doctors talking over me, having an oxygen mask forced on my face, the beginning of an ambulance ride, fear, pain. Much of it is a haze.

Most of the children who arrive at the hospital as I did for their initial diagnosis, in *acute diabetic ketoacidosis with renal complications,* never live to go home. The first hospital couldn't handle the severity of my condition, so I was sped in an ambulance eighty miles to the closest Nationwide Children's Hospital in Columbus, Ohio. I arrived in a coma and was placed in ICU. My doctor, a pediatric endocrinologist, afterward said to me that if I had arrived at the hospital any later that I would have died.

My family was saddled with the horrific financial burden of raising a diabetic child. I was the youngest of four children, which later increased to five. The logistical and emotional toll was even higher than the financial one. Measuring all foods. Reading all ingredients. Adjusting medications for me when my life was in danger. Learning about every aspect of a disease they personally would never experience. Enduring the personality and heath fluctuations that occur, day in and day out, as my blood sugars swing from high to low and back again. All day, every day.

Within a short time I was doing much of my management essentially on my own. I learned to make important discretionary decisions about my care and learned how to speak to doctors like an adult. To speak like an adult, I needed to be educated about my disease, to pose appropriate questions. To understand my doctor's reasoning behind this approach or that, I also had to learn to be assertive and to ask many, many questions. My doctor was there to help me, advise me on the best course of action, not to tell me what to do. I would, and still do, take advice and make a decision about how to approach a situation based on what I know in conjunction with what my doctor knows. I learned to take an active role in my care and to be my own advocate. Being an informed patient is a fine art. Those were good skills for a child to acquire in preparation for living successfully with a chronic, incurable disease. I was set on a plan to see my endocrinologist, discuss problems and develop new approaches every three months or so—for the remainder of my life.

A common, less-talked-about complication of T1D, called *hypoglycemia unawareness,* is also part of my condition. Twenty-four years after I was first diagnosed I still suffer from this complication. Essentially, the more you experience the symptoms of low blood sugar—shakiness, sweating, disorientation, and palpitations—the less your body and mind can recognize them. I usually do not get any of those warnings when I am nearing a dangerous blood sugar. My body does not warn me that I am impaired and need help. The lower I get, the more the danger. Because I am diabetic, the tighter my "control," the more likely I am to experience hypoglycemic events. This is because if you aim for a blood sugar of 80 or 90, which is ideal, if there is any error in estimation in your carbohydrate content versus the insulin you have given for that carbohydrate (even a very small miscalculation), you may end up with low blood sugars.

After a divorce, readjusting to living by myself was taking a large toll on me. I had been struggling with *nocturnal hypoglycemia* (low blood sugars while asleep), a problem that seemed to be getting worse. I was even awakened by the fire department once while stuck in a hypoglycemic state. The firemen probably saved my life. I followed diligently my doctor's orders, but just seemed to be having a worse and worse time with my diabetes, and my two other immune-mediated diseases. The other illnesses also affect blood sugar so I found it very difficult to know where to start.

The stress peaked in 2009. I was hospitalized in an ICU for a week with diabetic ketoacidosis after my insulin pump got ripped off my skin while I was asleep. Adhesives do not stick well to my skin and this was not the first time this had happened. Sadly, this time I did not wake up for many hours as the process of DKA took hold. When I finally woke, I was so lethargic that I could hardly move. I started profusely vomiting. I couldn't walk: my body felt like it was made of bricks. I crawled to the fridge to get new insulin, a new infusion set, and a new cartridge. I reloaded my insulin pump, and started trying to get my situation under control. When there was no downward motion in my blood sugar level, I tried insulin shots. I tried to force water down my throat. I tried to be level-headed because I needed to get my blood sugars down immediately. I was unsuccessful. The pain was mind-blowing. I started to have extreme chest pain so I called my friend Bob for help. He came to get me when I decided that I needed to go to the ER. I was concerned that I might be too critical, might be dying. In fact, I was. The small act of having an infusion set rip out came with a hospital bill larger than the amount I made that year, let alone the cost to my health. It was the final straw. I had to find something that would work.

***

I felt that I was just living on borrowed time. These events were happening far too frequently. My sister helped me look for options, new approaches or products out on the market that might work for me. Many of the products seemed good, but not versatile enough for my situation. We read about diabetic alert dogs and I investigated more. There were several facilities training dogs for that, but when I called, many of them left me with unanswered questions, hesitations, sticker shock, and a sour taste in my mouth. There was also a recurrent theme: they only wanted to train service animals for children. This struck me as strange since those same children will one day grow to be adults who will still need the help of a service dog. I even had my own pet dog, Maya, a six-year-old terrier mix, evaluated to see if a trainer thought she could be trained to provide this help for me, but I realized that I needed a dog hard-wired for this kind of work.

After much research and many phone calls, my sister found a mention of Wildrose and Mike Stewart from an article published in 2009 in *Forbes* magazine. We next learned of the Wildrose diabetic alert dogs. The idea of a service dog that could wake me from sleep for low or high sugar levels sounded promising. A dog that could be trained to bring me a glucometer or a juice when I was unable to move. A dog that could alert me of blood sugar problems when I was unaware, and that could return much of my sense of independence. A dog that could be versatile enough to fit into my less-than-typical life.

I was traveling often to see friends in Chicago. I had finally started churning out paintings again, which was like a breath of relief after the worst creative block I had ever experienced. I was biking and hiking with my dog, Maya. I was working all night and trying to take advantage of available things to do in the daylight. In the midst of my overwhelming medical problems, I was still alive and kicking. I felt hopeful. So I made some calls about a dog.

My first conversations with Cathy Stewart and Rachel Thornton were candid. I tried to be as direct as I could be about why I needed their help. I talked about what unawareness was like, and about how I was very concerned that I was going to die in my sleep. About how—regardless of what I seemed to do—I was still experiencing very dangerous blood sugars, often. I expressed my hope that one of their diabetic alert dogs might be the mediating factor that could help me get back in control of what seemed to be escalating medical problems. Cathy, and later Rachel, talked about the dogs, the kind of things they do, the owner's big commitment and responsibility, the length of training, the process of getting one, the estimated cost of training... They also stressed the fact that diabetic alert dogs are not and will never be perfect, but will be a new tool to use.

***

In March of 2010, the dog that would be trained for me was born at Wildrose. She was a very small British Labrador pup from a pairing of dogs named Whiskey and Katie. I named her Juniper after the plant, which has been used to treat diabetes by Native Americans for ages. They emailed me a picture of her, a roly-poly-looking ball of yellow fluff with oversized ears and soft eyes. Over the next year I kept in contact with Robinsons, the family who was raising and training Juniper. We discussed my needs and what they would be able to accomplish through training. My daily life is complicated, and fitting in a service dog would be difficult. I live in a big city and am a third-shift worker at an animal ER. I avidly travel to even larger cities by bus, train, car, or plane. I ride bikes and often attend music or art venues. It was daunting for me to contemplate how Juniper could fit my lifestyle. Would I have to adjust my life to her? Would she adjust to me? Or would we both modify together?

I tried to think proactively to prepare for life with a service dog. I thought about my daily life, to figure out how I might react with a dog at my side: at work, the grocery store, a library, the subway, a music venue, on my bike, on busy streets, around loud city sounds, at a thrift store, at an art museum, etc. I thought about protecting her feet, especially in the city, from glass and heat on city streets. I purchased Ruffwear dog shoes for rugged hiking. To protect her hearing at music venues or other loud events, I purchased Mutt Muffs, which are designed to protect the hearing of dogs that ride in plane cockpits. I purchased a top-of-the-line collapsible bike dog trailer from Pet Ego, which would, I hoped, enable me to continue riding my bike while in the city.

Over the course of the year I had many conversations about many service-dog-related things—with everyone. I had a bit of a challenge getting everything in order with my landlord and my workplace, in preparation for getting Juniper. My naïve impression of how things would go—should go—was just that, naïve. I tried to raise enough money to pay for the cost of Juniper's training. This was very difficult for me. Let's say from this experience I have learned to really put my money where my mouth is. If I think something is a good thing, I will invest in it. I found asking for donations humbling. My friend who had taken me to the hospital in 2009 had a good idea of what death from diabetes might look like, and so was kind enough to organize a music benefit for me. He was able to make connections and get a lot of local musicians together to do a punk rock benefit to help cover Juniper's cost. They donated the proceeds of entry to the show and the funds made from a raffle directly to the cost of training Juniper. Plus, the benefit was fun and full of awesome people and music. All of the rest came from my family and from a few friends.

I made plans to make several visits to work with Juniper and to train with one of the Wildrose trainers. Prior to bringing her home with me, I attended three diabetic alert dog workshops. The first time I saw Juniper I knew she was going to be a handful. She was lean and had a wild, happy expression on her face, as if she had a lot going in her head. The first time she saw me I think she knew who I was. She seemed to recognize my smell and she started wagging her whole body. At our first meeting, the trainers taught me the basics of handling a dog the Wildrose way. They showed me how to hold the leash, how to give a command, and how to correct a misstep, and then I tried it on my own. They corrected me as I went. By the end of the first day, I was fully engrossed in learning about this awesome pup and was highly intimidated by the things I would have to modify about myself: my tone of voice, my posture, my overabundance of eye contact... I was very anxious, because I needed this venture to work well. No amount of preparation could have prepared me for my first few months with Juniper. It was like having a new baby without the ability to really be separated from her. The first night she stayed with me in Oxford, Mississippi, after picking her up from Wildrose, she was a high-strung, wild thing, unable to settle down. I tried the "turn off," and then tried it again. From this experience I gained a sliver of insight into how hard this life was going to be. I think Juniper did not know what she should do, being surrounded by my ever-fluctuating scent. Although she had been exposed to several diabetics, none of them were diabetics like me. She alerted like a beast. I had no idea that I was fluctuating that much. I was always dropping too low. I would correct. I would eat. I would adjust my basal level and I was still erratically swinging from high to low. It was the beginning of new epiphanies about my disease. Juniper was giving me real information that I could use immediately. It was a scary undertaking. I was unsure how this new approach would unfold, so I started graphing the blood sugars.

Our first night together was terrifying and overwhelming for her and for me. The second night was much better. Juniper broke her place command, grabbed the bringsel from under my pillow and furiously nuzzled my face, then jumped on the bed, waking me up. She was so excited she was practically hopping over me. She gave me two nocturnal alerts, waking me up for a low and then for a high after my infusion set ripped out. I was so pleased with her alerts. I was reassured in a way that I can't articulate. I had confidence that this would work for my situation. We stayed through the rest of the diabetic alert dog workshop and then headed out.

***

As I left the Wildrose facility with Juniper, I felt good. We began our cross-country drive back home in Ohio to start a life together there. Several hours later, she alerted for me when I was driving. I pulled off, checked my blood sugar, and saw that it was low. I had already eaten my stash of low snacks, so I decided to just pull off at the next available spot to get additional food. I still had a little time before I was truly hypoglycemic, but I was dropping.

In Tennessee, I pulled off at a gas station and went in with Juniper. This was my very first time entirely on my own. The clerk started yelling at me that no pets were allowed. I told him that she was not a pet, that she was a service dog. I told him that she was allowed to accompany me, according to the Americans with Disabilities Act of 1990 (ADA). He demanded an ID. I explained that it is against federal law to ask or require that. I told him that I was having a medical emergency and that I needed to purchase food. He scoffed at me and asked what was wrong with me? I told him that it was illegal to ask that and it was rude to ask that. I reiterated that I was having a medical emergency and needed to purchase food. I reiterated that by federal law my dog was allowed to accompany me. He told me to get out of his store. I told him that he could not discriminate against me based on my disability. I gave an example of what most people are familiar with: a seeing-eye dog. This clerk told me that the blind leave their dogs at the door. I was so frazzled that I didn't know what to do. I needed food. I called the police.

The officer who arrived told me that even though this gas station served the public, that it was not covered under the ADA because it was privately owned. The officer told me that if the clerk didn't like how I looked he could refuse to serve me. I told him that the ADA does cover private businesses and that the clerk was in violation of federal law. I gave the police officer examples and I told him that I was having a medical emergency and that I needed food. He asked what was wrong with me. I told him that he was not allowed to ask me about my disability, that the clerk was required by law to allow my service animal to accompany me, and to allow me to purchase my food. I told the officer that either he could arrest me or that the clerk could sell me the food. The clerk angrily rang up the bill for the cost of the food. I ate and waited until I was okay to drive and then continued my drive home. I was so shaken by the lack of education of the clerk and police officer that I didn't really want to stop anywhere after that.

In Kentucky, I had to stop again and heard store employees talk loudly about Juniper and me. I told them that she was a service animal and that federal law guaranteed her the right to accompany me. They just continued talking about us as I sat down and ate in this restaurant. I still had several hundred miles to go, so I sucked it up and continued.

Once I got home, I had to go the grocery store to get a few essentials. I gave myself a liberal pep talk and went in. I went to get my items and had several clerks "ooh" and "ahh" about the pretty dog at my side. No one bothered me or even asked about her.

These three experiences gave me a lot of insight into how my life had changed overnight with the acquisition of my service dog. I thought a lot about what I should do with this big strange experience. How should I deal with this information? Did I handle the situation properly? Should I do something differently next time? Who I should contact about it? Should I file a Department of Justice complaint or try to talk to the responsible parties first? The week I got back, I tried to write down the incidents so I didn't lose details. I called the Department of Justice to inquire about filing a complaint. I decided that I would attempt to follow up with the owner of the gas station, but was given the runaround by the same clerk when I called. Researching a little bit, I attempted to contact the owner to make him aware of the situation. I called the store's oil supplier to make them aware also. The supplier was very apologetic and gave me more information to contact the owner. I made an official complaint there. I called the police chief of the city where this happened and asked him to educate his officers about the major civil rights law—only to be told the chief was also unfamiliar with the Americans with Disabilities Act of 1990. I explained the ADA to him. I told him that his officer's actions could have cost me my life. He promised to follow up with the Department of Justice and with his staff. He told me he would. I decided that the local grocery store that I went to that day was going to be the only one that I would go to for a while. I wanted to put my money where my mouth was. I stopped in and told the manager that the good response from employees really makes a difference to people who have special needs.

In retrospect, I learned a few good things:

Many people will not understand public access law even if you explain it.

Follow-up is important, whether in complaint or in appreciation. If I don't follow up, I am leaving that same bad situation for someone else to experience.

I always give myself much more time to accomplish a task now, because someone might stop me with questions.

Having a DAD is a civil rights issue, and I might have to stand up for my rights at times.

***

My life with Juniper adjusted quickly as routines were established. Juniper wakes me by moving from her place, which is beside my bed, to in *my* bed and I give her a belly rub. The belly rub is all-important in her eyes, so I only give it as a reward for nocturnal alerts, which are all-important in my eyes. I wear the bringsel on me while asleep. Juniper jumps into my bed, tugs the bringsel and licks my face. It is hard to stay asleep with a forty-pound dog walking on you.

When I wake up, I go through the same routine with her giving me the bringsel and finding my meter. I tell her, "Let's check." I see what the reading is and we go from there. When it's correct, I rub her down, give her much praise, and let her snuggle up to me, which she really loves. She quickly became a snuggly dog.

***

Alerting is a frenzied event in our house. It happens at any time of the day or night. Because I work at night, we get up to get our day started in the afternoon. When Juniper first bounces off her place, she always has a hard time staying at heel, but she has learned to correct herself. She ambles a step ahead, realizes that I have stopped, and jumps back to be beside me again with a goofy expression indicating that she wants me to hurry up. The first walk of the day is very slow, step by step, for this reason. The faster she goes, the slower I walk.

Juniper and I do some kind of activity to start our day. Rally-type activities—walking in circles, or random sits, or commands given twelve times during our walk—energize her. I try to include them in many of our daily exercises, because they engage her brain and remind her to pay attention to me. I like to keep her on her toes. After taking care of the rest of the household—my additional pet dog, Maya, and two cats, Ludo and Sake—we go on to face the rest of the day.

I initially worried about how my bouncy Lab would get along with my other animals. They all get along great. The two dogs sit there like old ladies together, acknowledging, but not engaging, each other. Juniper, however, does seem to have an ongoing relationship with my cat Ludo. I often find them asleep together. It doesn't seem to affect Juniper's alerting ability, so I think it's okay, at least for our team.

I had wondered how Juniper would do working late at night on third shift, but she has adjusted well. I work in an ER for animals, so the day-in day-out distraction is very high. Sitting on a Kuranda bed in a hollowed-out place under a counter, Juniper wears a leash attached to a prong on the wall so she can get up but can't go too far. All night long she and I are having a conversation that no one else understands. I check in with her sometimes. Other times, I see her get up to sniff the air, so I glance at her and decide what her body language says, and we go from there. Sometimes I put the bringsel right beside her. Sometimes I wear it on me. I think the variety is good for her because it makes her focus on different things. Sometimes she will hop in place, waiting for me to come around the corner so she can grab the bringsel off my hip. My coworkers know to tell me if she grabs the bringsel off the wall or if she is acting antsy.

People constantly ask about her. I politely tell people that she is a service dog and that they should try their best to ignore her because getting attention from others really distracts her from doing her job. There are many questions, especially because sometimes she alerts me in the middle of doing something for a client. Usually this is met with amazement that Juniper can do something so important for me, so often times I am met with more questions. Since I work with the public, I try to educate people on good service dog etiquette.

My coworkers adjusted easily to her being there. I think it is still hard for some of them to not love on her the way they do with their own animals. They often say she has the softest, most beautiful eyes. It has taken a lot of education to get us all to a comfortable point. People see her Service Dog Vest, but don't read or process what the patches mean: "Do not distract—working dog." Fellow employees and people in general have seemed to think that this phrase means just "Do not touch her" instead of the more accurate "Don't talk, touch, pet, stare, or make noises at the working dog." Fine lines are sometimes difficult to convey.

People also ask the question, "Does she ever just get to be a dog?" I answer that she gets to be a dog all day every day, because she gets to do what her body and brain are hardwired to do—retrieve all day long for me. She also gets to go everywhere with me, so a dull day for her would be a very exciting day for any other dog: car, bus, train, plane, store, restaurant, bike, park, and lake. She has a good life, full of dog activities.

Prior to getting Juniper, I read many books on dog cognition to better understand how I could enrich her life. I have tried to observe her, judge how she is handling new situations, and adjust from there. I knew that her job would afford her no real time off. I also knew that I would have to be very consistent in how I interacted with her, so our relationship would be pretty rigidly structured. This felt like a bit of a dilemma for me, because although I needed her to work for me, I also wanted her to be a happy dog, with her own personality. After being in her company for a bit, I was relieved that her bold personality is not diminished at all by the structure, but instead shines through in it. The structure gives us a better ability to communicate with each other. The obedience training that we have built upon gives us a common language. I try to give her plenty of exercise, and good food in addition to the fun activities. We go on bike rides and hikes. We are even working on getting comfortable with kayaking. I want her to have the best that I can provide for her, because she works hard to keep me safe and healthy.

Since I am so busy at work, running around our facility, I decided to convert Juniper's commands into hand signs. This would afford me the ability to multitask and to tell her something at a distance, while I was finishing a call or handling a "life-or-death" situation with a client. Also, dogs communicate with each other with body language. We have signs for "sit," "stay," "leave it," "under," "here," "heel," "place," "Juniper," "watch," and "quiet." We practice with only the signs, only the verbal cues, or both, to keep it interesting for her.

During an alert I carefully observe Juniper's body language in order to evaluate what she is telling me with her expression and body posture. She has a particular facial expression with intense eyes—a predatory or engrossed look with her body fully tensed—when things are serious. She is persistent in that state.

I could put her back on place and she would come right back off, only to grab the bringsel again. When she is like that, she is the boss, and I listen to her.

Juniper is very accurate, even if it's not immediately obvious to me. For example, once she kept alerting me at close to normal blood sugar for several hours. I did not know why. I thought that it had to mean something so I started brainstorming. I figured out that she was alerting me because I was spilling ketones.

Your body produces ketones when it's breaking down fat for energy instead of using sugar. Usually this happens to a diabetic when there is not enough insulin in the body to use the sugar in the blood. Ketones form in the blood but will be *spilled* into the urine. This is a concern for a diabetic because ketones make you very sick. The larger the ketones are, the more the concerned you should be, because they can lead to DKA. Once I became aware that I was spilling ketones, I took steps to remove them from my body. I started drinking water to flush them out of my system. Once they were gone, she stopped alerting that way. Now, every time Juniper alerts me at a close to normal number, I will check to see if I am spilling ketones. Sure enough, she will be right.

✳✳✳

Juniper requires a lot of mental stimulation, so I try to keep her engaged and give her opportunities to work things out on her own. I try to give her problems to solve so that she is increasing her reasoning skills. Retrieving is an easy activity to make her think and build problem-solving skills. I always use it as a reward for good alerting throughout the day, not as exercise. I use three types of retrieves: a memory, a sight, and a blind.

In a *memory* retrieve, I place an item and leave it while walking. When we get a good distance away, I make her sit and be quiet. Once she settles and is focused, I will release her and let her go get it for me. I use memory retrieves often, especially with my glucometer. If I am at work and need to get something in another department, I will take Juniper with me, dropping my meter somewhere along the trek, and will give her time to notice. Then I will continue running my errand and will stop somewhere close to the glucometer. I will sit her down, telling her to quiet. Once she realizes what we are doing, she settles down and looks at me with intense, focused eyes. I tell her, "Find the meter," which is her release for that particular item, and she goes and gets it for me, even though I may have dropped it ten minutes prior. She runs back so pleased with herself, giving me her sharky expression—mouth fully agape, her body in a partial play posture, as excited as she could be. Once she presents it to me I praise her and then give her the "turn off" which is a hand cupped under the side of her face. This is a very important trained behavior. I use that same turn off after every alert to let her know the excitement is over now and it is time to be quiet and polite.

In a *sight* retrieve, I have Juniper sit quietly and I show her what I want her to retrieve. I tell her to watch, and walk away from her, placing the object somewhere far away. Usually, I use a ball, a meter, or a juice box. When I return to her and when she becomes quiet, I say her name, which is a release. She runs, as if it is what she is meant to be doing—fast. She finds it, gets it, and runs it back to me. She presents it and I praise her. I then give the turn off and we go back to normal. I recently had her do a sight retrieve in a pool. She loves water—ears up, prancing her feet. She doesn't like jumping into the water: she would prefer to wade in, so I was interested to see how she would work it out. She ran around the pool to a raft floating on the side. She tried to walk out onto the inflatable raft, which would have put her right next to the desired ball. However, the raft was too unsteady, so she ran back to me. I pointed to the steps down into the pool, so she ran down, swam past my ball, retrieved someone else's ball and my ball and brought them both back to me. Without mental stimulation and exercise she is much harder to handle.

She focuses on me best when she is actively engaged. Because of this, I try to work training into every little niche I can.

A *blind* retrieve is by far the most difficult of the three for Juniper. She has to use her brain, her memory, her sense of smell, and her sight to figure out where the item might be. I set this retrieve up the same as the others except that Juniper does not see where I put the item. I tell her what item I need, and release her. She searches until she finds the correct item. She runs it back to me galloping, happy at her success. I have been using this retrieve to encourage Juniper to search more than one room to find something. She goes to look in her familiar places and then has to expand her search.

Juniper is a vibrant, life-saving dog with a bubbly personality. She is not a perfect tool, does make errors, and has bad days like the rest of us, but with much patience we have grown into a very accurate, dynamic team. Juniper's ability to alert me has given me the help that I needed to get my diabetes back into good control. When she is concerned, I am now concerned. Because she is able to alert me so well, I have been consistently improving. With her alerts she has been able to wake me from sleep when I have been having dangerously low or high blood sugar. She has been able to make me aware when my blood sugar is beginning to become dangerous while I have been driving so I can pull over and treat the situation. And she has been adamant when I needed her to be, keeping on top of the situation. She endures my long work hours and strange shifts, while consistently alerting for my needs. She has played a vitally important role, enabling me to handle the burden of managing a very complicated disease. She has saved my life on many occasions. She ameliorates the issues that I have had with hypoglycemia unawareness, and I am so grateful to have her in my life.

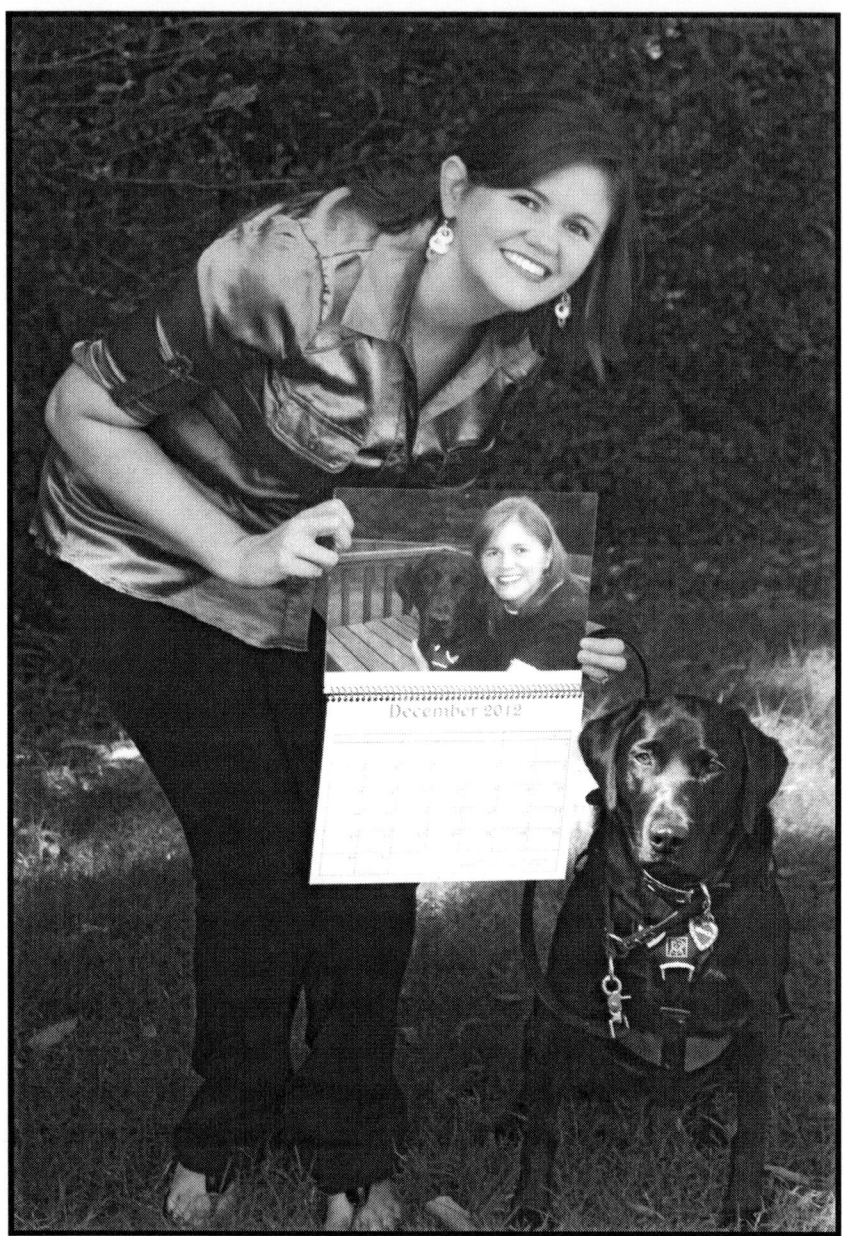

Sharon Stinson and Gracie.

Gracie and Sharon Stinson: Miracles and Misunderstandings

DURING MY SENIOR YEAR OF high school in Oxford, Mississippi, I began feeling tired and out of sorts. I started craving rich carbohydrate-loaded foods, but even though I ate nachos and tacos at Taco Bell nearly every day, I kept losing weight. After eating, I felt lethargic, weak, and extremely tired. I dropped down to 112 pounds. When I visited a doctor for a blood sugar test, he said that I was borderline diabetic. Not too concerned, he did not prescribe any medicine, but just told me to take care of myself.

Despite suffering through a miserable summer after graduation, in the fall of 1995 I moved into a Northwest Community College dorm apartment with two friends. I went to classes, and I began dating the man I would marry three years later. I tried to live a normal life. But my health was not normal. One of my friends, Katie, a nursing student, had several diabetics in her family and when she observed me, she said, "You have got to get checked for diabetes." So I went to another doctor, who shocked me with the news that I had full-blown type 1 diabetes.

At the time I did not really know what diabetes was because

there had been no history of diabetes in my family. I was very upset when the doctor told me I was diabetic, because all I could think of was the movie *Steel Magnolias,* in which Julia Roberts plays a young wife named Shelby, a diabetic who goes into a coma and dies.

So, when I was diagnosed, I thought, "Oh, my gosh, I am Julia Roberts. I am going to die right here and now. I am going to go into a coma and die."

I soon become educated about the disease. I began using an insulin pump to help regulate the high sugar count in my blood, but it was a huge struggle. My blood level changed so rapidly and often that I had great difficulty. Still, I went on with my life. I finished my studies and Jeremy and I married.

In the next several years I was in and out of the ICU and admitted to the hospital a lot. Frequently, I suffered diabetic seizures and we had to call ambulances to take me to the hospital. My husband and I joked that we paid for the hospital, because I went in so much.

For years and years my doctor said, "Oh, you're just brittle. There's just no hope of getting control over your glucose. You're just a brittle diabetic." I had so many problems controlling my sugar that for a time I fell into depression.

The years went on and I still had many, many problems. However, amid the tough times, I had some miraculous things happen in my life, too. During this time the doctor told me that I could have no children. That was such disheartening news for a young wife to hear, but as it turned out this news led to my first miracle after being diagnosed.

***

Ten years after my diagnosis, I continued having trouble controlling my sugar levels. I remember looking at my *People* magazine one day and seeing an article about a little boy with a German shepherd dog, a diabetic alert dog. I thought, *That is crazy!* I had heard of seizure alert dogs, and dogs that detect bombs and things like that. But I thought, *That's nuts, this can't be true.* But I read the article and something told me, *You need this dog, you need a diabetic alert dog.*

I called my husband and said, "We're getting a dog." I need to explain that we already had three Pekingese at the time. Naturally, Jeremy, said, "I don't think so." But after we talked about it some more, he said, "We'll think about it. Let's talk about it later." By his tone of voice I thought that he was blowing me off.

Quite the contrary. He went behind my back and began looking on the Internet for diabetic alert dogs. After some research Jeremy contacted a lady named Rachel Thornton, whose daughter has a diabetic alert dog named Mr Darcy. Jeremy said, "Rachel, my wife is diabetic and I really want to surprise her with a DAD for Christmas."

Rachel said, "If you want to give your wife a dog, you need to discuss it with her beforehand." She advised Jeremy that having a DAD requires a life-changing commitment. Rachel further explained that handling a diabetic alert dog is a lot of work. She concluded that it is a team effort and we both needed to be involved in the decision.

When Jeremy told me about his conversation with Rachel, I was so relieved and happy. A month later, in September, we met with Rachel. At first she tried to talk me out of it. Rachel said, "If you're not committed to this, it's going to fail. You have to be one hundred percent in. This is your time. This is your life. It's got to be a commitment."

But I was determined to get some help, and Jeremy and I both agreed to it. Rachel told me to call Cathy Stewart at Wildrose Kennels. As it turned out, I knew Cathy from Oxford many years earlier. I said, "Miss Cathy, we're ready. We want a puppy. We decided that we're going to train the dog ourselves, the Wildrose way, with help from your staff."

Cathy put us on the waiting list. Usually the waiting period to get a puppy is a year to eighteen months. Instead, we were confronted with another miracle. In November, just two months later, I got a call from Cathy.

"Sharon, there's a man here that doesn't want this puppy because she is the wrong color. Do you want her?"

I thought, "Are you kidding me, Lord?"

I told Cathy, "Of course, we want her. Right away."

Our puppy was born on November 3, 2009, the same day my father-in-law died of cancer at age forty-seven. To me, that was a confirmation from the Lord that this puppy was meant for us. I felt like my father-in-law was looking out for me.

Shortly after that phone conversation, Jeremy and I went to a diabetic alert dog conference at Wildrose, where we met many people who already had DADs. Mike demonstrated training techniques and Rachel showed scent-training strategies. We also gained practical information from other people that would be helpful as we began working with our dog.

***

On a gray, mid-December day, Jeremy and I drove to Wildrose and got Gracie. We named her that because she is my saving grace. She was just six weeks old. We brought her home and started training immediately: crate training, socialization, and obedience. Most people who receive DADs get them when the dogs are about two years old and have completed a DAD training regimen with professional handlers. However, some choose to get a very young pup and do the basic training themselves. Fortunately, because I live just a few miles from Wildrose, I could easily get help when I needed it.

Gracie was an exceptional pup. Within the first week that we had her, she started whining—this high-pitched, screeching whine that I had never heard from a dog. When I picked her up, she whined, smelled me, and licked my lips. I thought what she did was interesting, so I checked my blood sugar. Every time she did that and I checked my sugar, it registered over 200. We did not even train her to do that. She just smelled something on me. So, every time Gracie started to whine and lick my lips, we taught her to wave her paw. That's how we taught her to alert for high. Gracie has always been ahead of my meter with her alerts. Sometimes she's an hour ahead of my meter indicating a drop in my sugar level.

I remember one day when Gracie was urgently nudging me with her nose (our low-alert signal), I checked my blood sugar; it was 300, which is in the high range. But Gracie was nosing me. I thought this dog is nuts. I considered that she was merely seeking attention. However, a short time later when I checked, it had dropped to 60.

Training her to detect lows was more involved. When my blood sugar was low, at 75 or lower, I got a cotton ball, placed it in my mouth, and wet it with saliva. I could store several samples in Baggies in the freezer for two weeks. Whenever I wanted to train Gracie, I would take out a cotton ball, thaw it, and hide it somewhere in the house. Then, on command, I would allow Gracie to find the low. She would sniff it out, and we'd have a huge party and praise her. When she found it and offered the correct signal, we would give her peanut butter for her reward. For this training I just kept hiding it in different places in the house and send her to find it. Within one week, she started alerting me for lows.

Now, she wakes me up at night to alert me. One night she woke me up at two; I checked and was at 54. There are a number of instances when she has done unusual things to alert me. One Friday a few years ago Gracie and I accompanied my husband on a professional trip and checked into the Beau Rivage Resort in Biloxi on the Mississippi Gulf Coast. Our room was on the fourth floor of this very large casino-hotel. When we woke up on Saturday morning, Jeremy said to me, "Honey, sleep in. I'm going to take Gracie outside to go to bathroom."

So they went down the long hall and into the elevator and began going down. Gracie began to nudge him with her nose. He thought she was just misbehaving or acting strange in this new place. She kept insistently nosing him, so he took her back up in the elevator. When they got back up to the fourth floor and the elevator doors opened, Gracie ran down to our door. She knew which one it was. When Jeremy let her in, she went straight to my bed and jumped up next to me. I checked my blood sugar and it was 60. She had saved me again.

Another time, last spring, Gracie worked extra hard to get me help when I ignored her alert. I teach piano lessons to children after school, and Gracie and I were in the piano room at the Lafayette County Schools. I was sipping a Pepsi out of a large plastic bottle, just waiting with Gracie between lessons, the two of us alone in the room. Gracie began nosing me. Because I had just drunk the Pepsi, I told Gracie that I was okay, but she continued nosing me. When I ignored her, Gracie became more insistent. I thought she was just being bad. I tried to redirect her by telling her "sit," while holding her lead. She tore out of the room and went out into the building through a large roomful of over a hundred students, who were playing in after-school. She went straight to the two teacher supervisors and led them to my room. As it turned out, when I checked, my blood sugar was low. Because my sugar was low, I had not been thinking clearly at the time. Gracie had alerted others because I was not responsive.

Gracie alerted to other people, as well. Some DADs alert solely to their handler once they have been trained with that person. However, other DADs will alert to any diabetic that they come in contact with. Once, when my mother-in-law was visiting, Gracie got my meter and dropped it in her lap. My mother-in-law looked at me and said, "I don't have diabetes." I suggested that she go to her doctor and get checked out. When she did, her doctor found her blood sugar at 250. She has Type 2 diabetes.

Another time when Gracie and I were shopping in a clothing store, Gracie nudged another lady with her nose. I said, "Pardon me, but do you have blood sugar problems?" The lady said that she didn't, but that she had a doctor's visit scheduled soon and she would have him check. I gave the lady my telephone number and asked her to please call me after her doctor's visit. A few days later she called me. It was a Friday night. She said, "You won't believe this, but my doctor told me that I am diabetic."

***

I am passionate about educating people about diabetic alert dogs. I don't know how some diabetics manage without one. But having a DAD also brings with it some difficult issues. Two that I have faced are public access and obedience training.

One day, Gracie and I were grocery shopping in a large chain store in Oxford. I had shopped at this popular store several times before with Gracie, so I was startled when an overly assertive manager trainee approached and asked me to leave with Gracie immediately. She had her service vest on and I assured him that she was a service dog and was permitted to be in the store. But this aggressive manager-in-training followed us around store, harassing us, saying that we had to leave immediately. He claimed that he had checked with officials at the public health department and they had said that no dog was allowed in the store. He angered me to tears, making a scene in front of everyone, and escorting us out of the store. Later, I spoke to another employee, told him about the incident, and explained in detail the pertinent points of the Americans with Disabilities Act (ADA). The manager called me and said that he was sorry and that I could come back with Gracie. I encouraged the manager to educate his employees so that customers would not be mistreated as I had been. Later, the overzealous manager trainee called to apologize, but he never admitted that he had not really called the county health officials. Afterwards I called them myself and they assured me that they knew the law, had not talked to this person, and would never have told any businessperson otherwise.

As I said, I am passionate about diabetic alert dogs and I wanted to educate more people about public access laws, so I agreed to do an interview for the local newspaper. *The Oxford Eagle* ran a front-page story with pictures, presenting my story of working with Gracie as a service dog. The news story quoted city officials and emphasized the public access laws, spelling them out in detail, which was my purpose in doing the interview. I have also spoken to local groups, presenting my journey with Gracie in managing my diabetes and explaining to them the laws that make it possible for Gracie to be with me wherever I go.

***

Gracie, despite her foibles, was a blessing. Unfortunately, her story ended on a sad note. Gracie died prematurely. She suffered a freak, but all-too-common, home accident for children and pets: suffocating in a plastic bag. She saved my life so many times. I wish I could have saved hers. As all pet owners know, losing a family dog is losing a member of the family. Losing my DAD is doubly hurtful, because I lost my medical assistant as well as my constant companion. The Wildrose staff has been so graciously helpful. Cathy Stewart and Rachel Thornton provided me with a temporary replacement. Jeremy and I decided to raise and train a new puppy and we were blessed to get Maia, a seven-week-old. On the Fourth of July, 2013, Maia made her first real-time alert. She tried to jump at my mouth while sniffing like crazy and licking my lips. I checked my BG while she looked at me intently and it was 89 and dropping. YES! Good low!

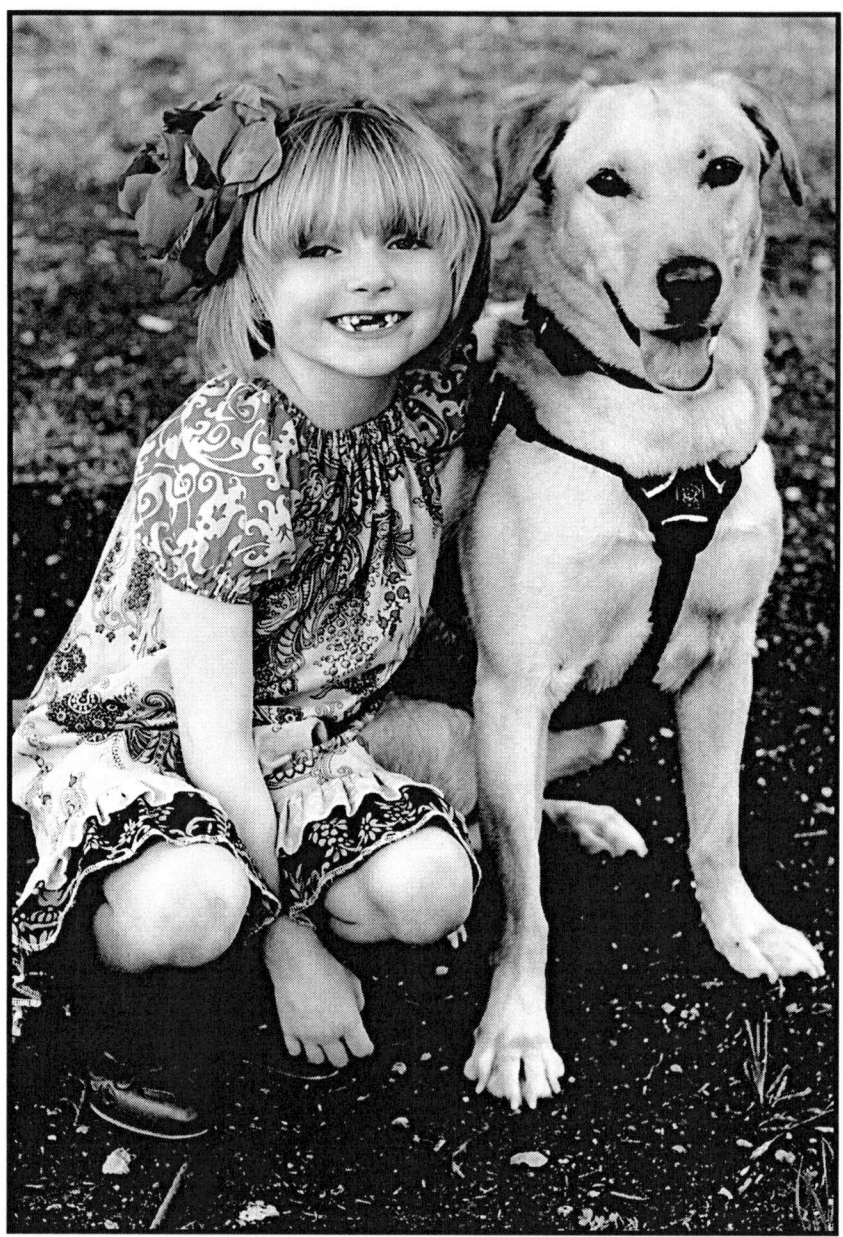

Lily Simonton and Charlie.

Charlie, Lily and Angie Simonton: Focus in School Settings

THE MONTHS AND WEEKS LEADING up to my daughter's diagnosis seemed like any other winter in Colorado, filled with childhood colds and viruses. Even though I had noticed changes in Lily's eating habits and she had become irritable, the doctors said not to worry, that it was normal for a child her age. I had noticed her soaking her diapers and drinking more than normal while still refusing to eat. I continued to see small changes, but nothing drastic, until I tried her new spring clothes on her. They were hanging on her little body and I remember thinking how I had really misjudged her size.

One April morning, we got up to get ready for our playgroup, Mothers of Preschoolers, but Lily seemed extremely tired. I remember thinking how she had gone to sleep so early the night before and that this was odd for her. She would not eat breakfast, or drink her usual milk or juice, and she continuously seemed to nod off. Something felt wrong. I decided to call my pediatrician's office to give me some peace of mind. They said since she didn't have a fever that I didn't need to bring her in. They guessed she probably just had a virus and suggested that I let her sleep.

Mother's intuition said differently. I quickly gathered my purse and keys, not even suspecting that I wouldn't return for days. As I picked Lily up to carry her to the car, she began to moan. It was as if her little body hurt for me to even touch her. Then I smelled the faint, fruity, ammonia-type smell. Five years later, I can still smell that strong odor as if it were just yesterday.

The drive down the pass from Woodland Park to Colorado Springs seemed like an eternity. Lily's moans became more frequent, her breathing became extremely labored, and it was almost impossible for her to stay awake. I remember her beautiful blue eyes disappearing from the review mirror for what seemed like minutes at a time. Arriving at Fort Carson's Evans Army Community Hospital, I frantically scooped Lily up and ran into the pediatrician's office. The smell was stronger and she was pale and limp. I assumed that they would quickly place me in a room, but I was wrong. I waited. I prayed.

Finally in a room, I was told the doctor would be in shortly. Time stood still and fear enveloped me. "Shortly" seemed like forever. In my heart, I knew something was really wrong, as Lily's symptoms continued to escalate. Something had to be done. I began screaming for a doctor to hurry. As he walked in, he took one smell and said the words that sadly changed our lives forever: "diabetic ketoacidosis." All I caught was "diabetic," but I knew. My dad had type 2 diabetes and was insulin-dependent, so I had an idea of our future. The attendants quickly whisked Lily to another room and pricked her finger—the first of a lifetime of finger sticks. The blood sugar meter read "HI," which meant nothing to me at the time. They explained that Lily would be transported to the Pediatric Intensive Care Unit at Memorial Children's Hospital and that we would be there for at least a week.

My body was numb as I watched Lily lying lifeless on the table and giving a nearly silent moan as they repeatedly stuck needles in her arm attempting to start an IV. The single tear that rolled down her face crushed my soul. For the first time, I could not fix this for her. I was powerless against a powerful, invisible disease. My daughter, Lily, had officially been diagnosed with type 1 diabetes. How could this be? My child? Why? *My daughter would require constant monitoring and care in order to live.* Over the following four years, Lily continued to push forward through endless finger pricks, IV site changes, highs, lows, tears, sleepless nights, and constant worry. Her little body constantly changes, which means her care is never the same. I soon realized that I needed reassurance that this "invisible disease" was under control and that I was doing everything possible to ensure Lily the best care. Being a single mom, I needed another set of eyes and ears—and a nose! We needed a diabetic alert dog. I had seen various articles on these dogs and had read what they could do for type 1 diabetics. Soon thereafter, I encountered a family with a DAD at a local Juvenile Diabetes Research Fund meeting. This family spoke highly about what their DAD brought to their family. I began researching every kennel offering reputable DADs that I could find. I was on a mission. I wanted to give my daughter the healthiest life possible. She deserved more, and diabetes does not sleep. It doesn't go away. It never takes a vacation. For me, there are always questions: Did I count those carbs correctly? What is her blood sugar? Is the meter right? Do I need to check it again? Did she get too much insulin or not enough? Does she need an extra snack before ballet? Is she sleepy because she is tired or is she low?

***

After researching many kennels, I found Wildrose Kennels in Oxford, Mississippi. When I called to inquire, I was quickly placed in contact with Rachel Thornton for information about the DAD program, the application process, and an actual account of what life was like with a DAD. I remember my first conversation with her. Rachel was the kindest individual and could truly understand my fear as a mother, because she had a diabetic daughter and a DAD. However, she gave me every reason why it might not be the best decision. She wanted me to fully understand that this dog was not a pet, but a highly trained service animal that would change my life forever. She suggested that attending a diabetic alert dog conference would be our next step in the process, where we could immerse ourselves in a weekend of activities with families with DADs. And we could actually work with a service animal.

So Lily and I set out for the DAD workshop in Colorado in July of 2010. That weekend changed my life. I remember my range of emotions. I was scared, and even questioned my decision to proceed. Everyone was honest about how hard it was, but also about how rewarding having a DAD could be. I knew that my situation was special—a single mom and kindergarten teacher with a three-year-old type 1 diabetic child needing a DAD to attend a school setting. Looking back, I know that they thought I was crazy. Certainly, I needed the right dog for the right child for the right situation. Our DAD would need to know Lily was his job and that he needed to work for me and, at school, for her teacher. Wow, a big order to fill! As Lily and I left the conference, Rachel asked me to continue to think about the commitment and sacrifice that was involved in having a DAD. After the experience with the other DAD families, my mind was made up. I wanted and needed a DAD for Lily.

I still remember the telephone conversation with Rachel as she told me that she had found us a possible match. "Charlie is this goofy, gentle giant with a sensitive soul," she said. When we finally met Charlie, I knew that Rachel could not have been more right.

We needed a strong, confident DAD that could handle an early-childhood environment. Charlie was to attend preschool with Lily in a classroom of fifteen to twenty children and then move on to public school. Being a kindergarten teacher, I knew this was a tall order. The level of obedience had to be impeccable. He had to withstand a high amount of energy, noise, and unpredictable behavior while staying focused on *his* girl. At our second diabetic alert dog conference in May of 2011, this time in Oxford, Mississippi, we had our first opportunity to meet Charlie and to gauge his compatibility with our family. When we got to the conference, we saw that Charlie's temperament was everything that Rachel had described. We studied how he interacted with our family. I knew Rachel was watching closely even from afar. I was over the moon and nervous all at the same time. During the workshop training sessions I practiced heelwork and place training with Charlie. After only a few hours, Charlie alerted to a fluctuation in Lily's blood sugar. I was overwhelmed, excited, and really couldn't believe he had alerted to my daughter in a room full of other diabetics.

During the conference weekend, Charlie also spent the night with us at the hotel and we continued to slowly integrate him into our routines. He was great. I began to see just what Rachel meant when she said he would change our lives. It wasn't just about Lily and her care, but now it was about Charlie's, too. For the first time, I needed to think about feeding and watering routines, taking him out to potty, dressing him in a service vest, packing him up with a mat and bringsel, and all this was just for a day's outing. There were so many variables in caring for a service dog, and I knew that I was just scraping the surface of what life would be like with a DAD. Upon leaving the conference, I felt good about Charlie and his dynamics with our family; however, I knew that Rachel needed time to think over all the issues. She later called to say that he would be coming to Texas in June. We had a month to get ready for our newest family member.

Rachel brought Charlie to us and helped us to get acclimated. She stayed with us for five days while giving us the ins and outs of how to best integrate Charlie into our lives. We went to some of our most frequented places, including Lily's preschool. Rachel shared many ideas of how she felt the school setting should look and how I could integrate Charlie into the classroom. We both knew that school was going to be the big hurdle to cross. Of course, Charlie eventually filled those shoes wonderfully. Has it been easy? No. Our journey has been filled with much happiness, but many unforeseen tears, as well.

✳✳✳

Preschool life with a service dog presented many challenges. Consistency in handling was hard to maintain. Lily was obviously too young to handle Charlie completely on her own so Charlie looked to me for guidance, but when at school, he looked to her teachers. In a preschool setting, Lily had up to three teachers in a single day, which meant that Charlie would have to alert to many individuals. Training the teachers Charlie's commands and understanding the process of his alerts proved to be the hardest. Charlie's commands had to be precise and consistent, with the right tone and a slow, calculated tempo.

Beginning the month before school, I began taking Charlie into the school setting, allowing him to get familiar with the level of noise, activity, and what it would be like to follow Lily in a setting outside our home. We began with small increments working up to longer times. Once school began I would sit at the back of the classroom and watch Charlie interact with Lily, observe how the other children interacted with him, and see how he maintained steadiness in such an active environment. The children in the class did well after I explained why Charlie was in the classroom, what type of service Charlie performed, and that their responsibility was to not interact with him. In fact, training the children was the simplest of my tasks.

For the parents and staff, I wrote a letter explaining Charlie's role as a service dog and providing service dog etiquette. This was a hard task, for people are intrigued by dogs. Most people have the need to interact, touch, or talk to dogs regardless of the situation. But if every parent or staff member spoke to or attempted to interact with Charlie, they would be distracting his focus from Lily, and I would need to correct. All of these things could cause Charlie to miss making alerts and lose focus on his job, monitoring Lily's blood sugar level.

At the beginning of school, Charlie was working beautifully, catching shifts, making alerts, and keeping focused while I sat at the back of the room. Things seemed to be progressing as expected. However, getting teachers to master the level of consistency with his commands proved difficult. Most people have pets, not service animals, so they don't understand the extreme calculation of a command. Unfortunately, I will always take Charlie and the level of his training ten times more importantly than someone outside our family. My wish is for everyone to grasp the importance of Charlie's presence in Lily's life and just what he does for her.

During the first month that Charlie was at school with Lily, I began to see bits and pieces of his training unravel. First, his nighttime alerts stopped. He had been alerting consistently four to five times a night and now, abruptly, he ceased. I couldn't pinpoint why, but I knew it was due to something happening at preschool. Next, I noticed him missing alerts at home and even showing unpredictable behavior in public. I knew that after "pickup" each day I would need to go through several training exercises with Charlie before heading to the store or running an errand. He just seemed "off" or unsteady when commands were given. Also, his chain of alerts seemed to be breaking down. He had been trained to alert by bringing me a bringsel. However, now instead of retrieving the bringsel each time, he would follow me around the house just staring at me. He looked lost, as if he didn't know what to do. I spoke to Rachel on the phone. We both felt that removing Charlie from the situation was best until another trainer could come assess the situation at preschool. We decided to take him to a friend's house for several weeks. Sarah Wilson had a T1 daughter, Faith, and a DAD, Ruby, who was Charlie's littermate. Leaving Charlie was a very hard decision and it devastated Lily and me, but I knew it had to be done to save our DAD and his training. That seemed like the hardest two-and-a-half weeks of our lives. Once again, fear set in. Lily's numbers were all over the place and we experienced several extremely bad lows.

Beth, a Wildrose volunteer and one of Rachel's daughters, arrived in September and assessed the situation at school for seven full days. She attended preschool with Lily and Charlie each day and watched how he interacted and reacted to situations. She made keen observations and took notes, videos, and photographs. She regularly communicated with Rachel and other Wildrose staff members and proved to be a vital link in restoring Charlie to a high level of proficiency.

Charlie was the first DAD placed in an early-childhood environment, so these were uncharted waters. I knew there would be setbacks, but I would not accept failure. We had to try again.

To rectify the problems we had to retrain even the smallest details. First, we had to review service dog etiquette with all of the people involved. We sent another letter and Beth spoke with the teachers interacting with Charlie and Lily. Many found it so hard to understand *do not pet, touch, or talk*. Retraining all not to place their hands out for Charlie to sniff, and not even to speak to him was so hard for many to understand. Next on the agenda was finding the best scenarios for Charlie to have success in the classroom. Where to place him during the lessons? How would he transition to the playground? How to have consistency in alerting to Lily? Teaching consistency was the key.

By the time Beth left, the situation improved. I felt good and knew that Charlie was the right DAD for the job, but I also realized that it was out of my hands. The preschool staff had to be consistent and truly watch Charlie and Lily as "one" for this to work. For a few weeks, it did work, but then little things started to unravel again. Upon pickup one day, I stood outside the classroom door and watched Charlie attempt to alert the teacher. She missed the alert and quickly put him back on place in his designated spot on his cot. I couldn't believe my eyes—the teacher hadn't even recognized the alert of grabbing the bringsel from Lily nor did she tend to my daughter's medical need. Instead, she shut him down. As I continued to watch, he attempted to alert again and the teacher told him to return to place for a second time. Once I walked into the classroom, Charlie took the bringsel from Lily and brought it to me. We quickly checked and realized Lily's blood sugar was high. I looked at the record of her sugar levels on meter; I spoke with her teacher and began asking questions. The teacher told me that Charlie may have alerted her, but that "he" was not her priority.

At that moment, I realized that Charlie and Lily were not in the right environment.

I decided to move Lily and Charlie to a different teacher and retrain again. This was not a completely new teacher: Lily had had her two years prior, so she had knowledge of diabetes and the severity of Lily's condition. However, the children in that classroom were an entire year younger than Lily. Lily immediately missed her friends and being with children her own age. And I know Charlie picked up on her unhappiness. For the first time ever, Lily did not want to go to school. She begged to stay home and just wanted to be with her other friends. I couldn't make it right. I had to make the decision that was best for her *and* Charlie. The move was difficult, but it paid off. They strengthened as a team.

***

I truly believe it is hard for people outside of the family to understand the gravity of diabetes and then to understand the level of care and security these amazing dogs provide. Charlie saves Lily's life every day. He is so connected and in tune with her that it is amazing to watch. He loves *his* girl. On just another normal day at preschool in the late fall, Lily and her classmates were taken to a room at the other end of the school to hear a guest speaker. Charlie was left alone in the classroom. Lily's blood sugar was checked before she left to hear the speaker. She had just had a snack so the situation seemed to be under control. Lily's teacher ran back to the classroom a few minutes into the program, and Charlie was on his cot with a large, dried starfish from the science center in his mouth. She was very unhappy, scolded him, and returned the starfish to its place on the science table. She left Charlie and the classroom once again to return to the program. About fifteen or twenty minutes later she returned to the classroom, finding Charlie with the starfish in his mouth once again. This time a few arms were missing from its fragile body as Charlie held it tightly in his mouth while sitting on his cot. He had probably been holding it in his mouth for quite some time. The teacher scolded him again and took the starfish to the front office.

Luckily, the manager felt this was not typical of Charlie's behavior and decided to check on Lily in the program. Thankfully, she did because Lily's blood sugar had plummeted. Charlie's odd behavior had just saved Lily's life. Not only was Lily in the other classroom, but also so was the bringsel. Charlie was in an empty, closed classroom without his girl or bringsel. So he used his keen sense of smell to find the last thing that Lily had touched during center time. Lily had played with the starfish all morning long in the classroom prior to going to hear the guest speaker. What seemed to be naughty behavior was Charlie's way of telling the teacher to check his girl.

Charlie is very good about finding Lily's stuffed animals

or the last thing she touched if he is serious about alerting, especially if he thinks you are ignoring him or if it is at night. My favorite alert is seeing his sweet face holding blue bunny at two in the morning to give me an alert. Through pure exhaustion I can see a true miracle.

Once, Lily's preschool had a parent's night out so that we could Christmas shop. I took advantage, but felt that Charlie should not stay at the school because Lily's normal teachers were not there and they would be combining classrooms. So I did some shopping, picked Charlie up, and headed home to unload and eat dinner before heading back out for more shopping. Once we were home, I fed Charlie and he settled in for some downtime and a relaxing evening "off the job," which doesn't happen often for him. Things were uneventful other than Charlie having a few dreams while catching a nap. I then heard him becoming restless on his cot and noticed him getting off place to come towards me. I didn't say anything because I was curious as to why he would be getting off place when Lily was at preschool over six miles away. He soon began bumping my hand with his nose... one, two, three times. He then turned and retrieved the bringsel from the basket. I starting worrying about Lily because Charlie was so accurate and I had heard of remote alerts and stories of DADs alerting from crazy distances even though their person was not in sight.

I called the preschool and asked them to Check Lily's blood sugar. She was 173 with insulin on board. Hmmmm... great number, but Charlie was still pacing and alerting. Charlie is very persistent if he thinks you are not listening to him. So we jumped in the car and went to get our girl. Sure enough, I rechecked Lily thirty minutes later and it was 209. Good high, Charlie! We got in the car and before we drove away, he gave another alert. I rechecked, and 282. Whooohooo! Charlie gave another alert once we got home and rechecked. Lily was up to 317 forty-five minutes later.

Charlie is usually about forty-five minutes ahead of the meter. But how could this be? They were so far away from each other. I checked over Lily's numbers for the evening, what she had eaten, and how much insulin she had been given. I realized that Lily had not been given insulin after her dinner that evening, so Charlie was truly on the job.

Charlie has become just as important as Lily's insulin pump—part of her life support. I really didn't know how much Charlie would change our lives. Since getting Charlie our lives changed again, but in an entirely different light. I now have hope. I have security. We have love. Charlie is the most amazing dog that I have ever encountered. He is our guardian angel. We incorporate Charlie into every aspect of our lives: school, vacations, grocery shopping, ballet recitals, doctor's appointments, birthday parties... He brings such joy to our lives no matter the situation. Lily has a new playmate and friend. He is always there. He is consistent. He provides her a sense of security that she does not have with her disease. Diabetes is so unpredictable and Charlie is just the opposite.

Rarely have I chosen to not bring him along and crate him at home. We depend on Charlie's alerts. The few times that I have made the decision to crate him, we have felt disjointed. Charlie and Lily are connected and he knows she is his job and she knows he looks after her. For a successful DAD team, they must be immersed into every situation and become one. When we recently took a trip to Sea World, Charlie was amazing, and he gave us many wonderful memories. Seeing Charlie alert to Lily's blood sugar in an environment filled with people and numerous distractions was amazing. Sea World was hot, filled with many kids and adults that were not used to seeing a service dog, much less a service dog in shoes. It also presented different smells and noises, 3D movies, tanks filled with dolphins and whales and much more. Yet he was consistent, obedient, and kept his focus on Lily.

As I go through each day with Lily, Charlie, and diabetes, I often think of our journey and how we were brought together. When I ask myself why we were chosen to have diabetes, I simply remember this: If nothing ever changed, there'd be no butterflies. We had to experience diabetes to have Charlie.

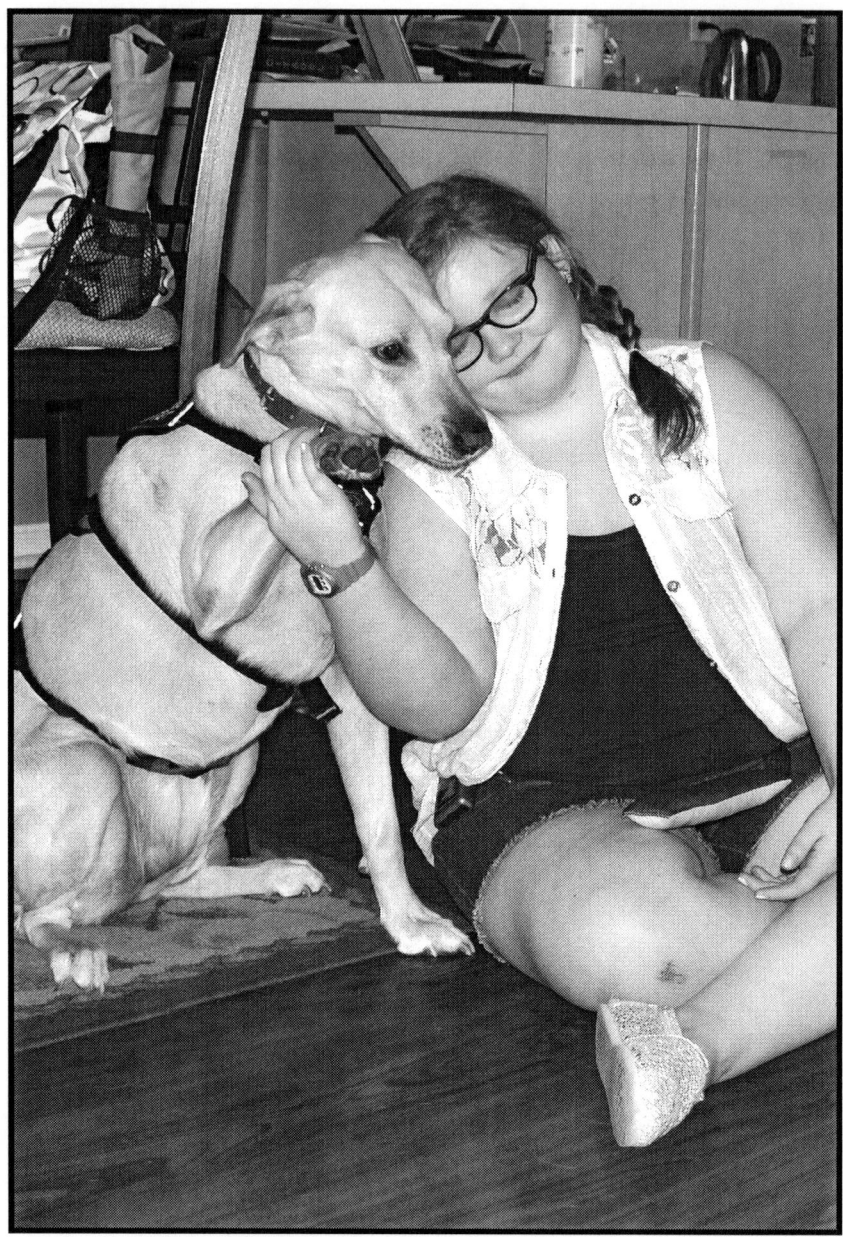

Keeper and Anna Grace Berry.

Keeper and Kitty and Anna Grace Berry: Our Journey

OUR SWEET ANNA GRACE WAS diagnosed with diabetes at the young age of four. As a parent, you always know when something just isn't right with your child. Anna Grace had been extremely thirsty, uncharacteristically tired and her lips were sticking together. Anna Grace's Daddy, Tim, was active duty Air Force and gone on another trip. I took her to Andrews Air Force Base Pediatrics because of an odd rash that I wanted evaluated. Her urine was tested and we were sent home with some cream. A few hours later, I received a call telling me to take her in for blood work because there was sugar in her urine. I didn't know what that meant. I brushed it off as non-urgent and decided I would wait for my husband to get home in a few days and have him join us for an unpleasant blood draw. The pediatrician called several times telling me that I had to get her in for blood work, but without telling me why. In a few days, Tim came home and off to the military hospital we went. The pediatrician met us at the lab, so we knew it was serious as we waited for the results. The doctor led us into a room and said those words that no parent wants to hear: "Your daughter has juvenile diabetes."

The pediatrician said we had to take Anna Grace to a major hospital immediately and, if we promised to go straight to Walter Reed Medical Center, she wouldn't call an ambulance. *An ambulance? Really?* We were bewildered.

We drove to Walter Reed, the Army's flagship hospital, located in Bethesda, Maryland, and were met by many people in masks and military uniforms. Anna Grace was severely dehydrated and they said that starting an IV was urgent. However, finding a vein in her tiny pale arms was nearly impossible. Several nurses and doctors held her down while she screamed, "Mommy! Daddy! It hurts! It hurts!" It was heart-wrenching, scary, and confusing. At this point, we didn't truly understand the turn our life was about to take. We didn't understand the seriousness of Anna Grace's condition or the disease. All we knew was that our baby was terrified and hurting. Anna Grace was sobbing on the gurney and looked paler, sicker, and weaker as the minutes crawled past.

Out of nowhere, a man appeared in full black military gear. He was fully armed and looked very intimidating. He knelt next to Anna Grace's bed and started whispering in her ear. He spoke very calmly, very softly to her. He sang to her and prayed with her. He calmed her sobbing little body and the nurses were finally able to get a line started. They administered her first dose of life-saving insulin. The color started coming back into her face and her lips started looking more normal and less like a parched desert. The unnamed man stayed with Anna Grace— and us. We exchanged casual, meaningless pleasantries and thanked him for his time. He held Anna Grace's hand, made her laugh, and comforted her and us with his presence. This was one of the first of many strangers with wings who entered our lives along this unimaginable journey. I never got his name or expressed my gratitude. After waiting for hours with our sick, tired, and terrified child, we were told Walter Reed couldn't accommodate Anna Grace and an ambulance was dispatched to take our baby girl to a children's hospital in Washington, D.C. We watched helplessly as her little body was strapped to the big black stretcher while too many people worked on her, checking vitals, drawing blood for labs, checking blood sugar, and measuring her input and output. It was all so hard to process and to understand. It was a nightmare. Little did we know it was only the beginning of the nightmare.

At Children's, Anna Grace was taken immediately to a room where more people with masks, more nurses, more doctors swarmed her bed checking vitals and lines and insulin dosages. An air of silent urgency hovered in the room. Concern covered the faces that met us. We were told that Anna Grace was very sick and in diabetic ketoacidosis. She would need insulin for the rest of her life to stay alive. What? Our child? Please God, NOT our child. They put Anna Grace on a constant drip of sodium chloride and insulin to gradually rehydrate her body and lower her dangerously high blood sugar. Her blood sugar reading after insulin was administered was a frightening 900. Normal for a child Anna Grace's age is about 80.

The initial education we received on how to manage diabetes was overwhelming. We were in a state of crisis. We were crammed in a tiny, hot hospital room where we hadn't had any sleep for days. How could we possibly be expected to manage all our emotions? Our family was changed forever in a moment. Anna Grace was still so tired, so thirsty, so pale looking, so sick. We were supposed to be able to understand, to know how to draw up insulin, measure dosages, count carbs, check blood sugar and give injections. It was so much to take in. It was too much to take in. After a four-day stay that seemed like a month, we were released to the world. We were told that we were "sufficiently trained." We were armed with phone numbers, protocols, meters, needles, insulin, charts and follow-up appointments. We went home exhausted, bewildered, worried and scared. How would we manage this disease? How would we keep our precious child alive?

I will never forget the very first time I pricked Anna Grace's finger to test her blood sugar and she screamed and cried, "Ow, Mommy! Why do you want to hurt me?" Hurting my child to keep her alive became a necessary evil. There are needles to check blood sugar levels, needles to administer insulin, needles for infusion sets attached to an insulin pump, needles for emergency glucagon. Most people fear needles, fear pain. Diabetics don't have the luxury of fearing needles.

When a child is diagnosed with a chronic disease, the whole family is diagnosed with a chronic disease. In the first six months, every moment is consumed with managing the disease. Everyone in the house becomes a nurse, a caregiver. You no longer take for granted the boring, normal days when you can go on spontaneous journeys unprepared. Your life is now forever tied to life-saving supplies that must accompany you everywhere. You arm yourself with knowledge on how to manage the invisible disease that the world thinks is "no big deal." You arm yourself with knowledge on how to keep your child alive. The first time you witness your child's blood sugar drop to a dangerous 20 and see her become incoherent, the first time you see your child's body overcome with a seizure due to a sudden, unexpected low, the first time you read about a child's life taken too soon by diabetes, you realize how dangerous and precarious this disease is. Failure isn't an option, so you research more and find every tool out there to help you battle this unwelcomed visitor. That's how we found out about diabetic alert dogs that were being trained to detect and alert their owners to changes in blood sugar levels. We were thrilled! Another set of eyes, another tool to help us protect our child.

We researched and researched and called and called. We read, we studied, and we read some more. We found many organizations that were unwilling to work with children and other organizations that had waitlists of years. We were frantic parents wanting to do everything within our power to help Anna Grace battle this disease. We found an organization that was willing to work with a child and proudly reported that it had a perfect success rate. We used our summer vacation time and funds to travel out of state. We were told we would train with our child's new lifesaving tool that had a proven record. We would learn how to successfully teach our new service animal to perform like a champion and save our child. We were armed with hope and a willing heart and set out on our first journey into the diabetic alert dog world. We reached out to family and friends to raise the thousands of dollars needed to fund this animal.

***

Our training was nothing short of a nightmare. We were paired with a sick dog that was much too small for Anna Grace and had no interest in being her dog, let alone her lifesaver. We expressed concerns to the organization on the very first day. We worked hard trying to mold the dog into a willing member of our family. We worked hard practicing the skills and commands and diabetic alerting we were promised would come. Each day was a miserable failure. Each day we lost hope. The final day of our training, after protesting endlessly to the owner, we were finally paired with a border collie mix with a vibrant and willing personality. She was sweet, obedient, and large enough to take care of Anna Grace. We were ignorant and desperate for a lifesaver and took the dog home, once again filled with hope.

After working for a year to train an alert, we came to the conclusion that the dog was unable to do diabetes work. We worked very hard to teach the dog to recognize the dangerous changes in Anna Grace's blood sugar. We called the organization, we begged for help. We received little and were left to figure it out on our own. We continued to research and read and try, but we knew deep in our hearts that even though this dog may have many good features, it would never be able to save Anna Grace's life. Failure wasn't an option. We felt betrayed and bewildered. How could an organization willingly take thousands of dollars from a child and promise to provide a tool that would save her life when they knew that was highly unlikely? Nevertheless, we still felt that our child's life would be improved and made safer with a diabetic alert dog, so our search continued.

Through our frustration, desperation, continued research, faith and prayer, we met another stranger with wings named Rachel Thornton. She shared our frustrations and wanted to help us find a better solution for Anna Grace. She made herself available to us and introduced us to Wildrose Kennels in Oxford, Mississippi. Rachel knew us only from phone calls and emails. She knew us only as another desperate family living the same nightmare that she had lived with her daughter, Abi.

At about the same time we were speaking with Rachel, Anna Grace had started showing gross motor delays. Doctors tossed around phrases about muscle disease and mitochondrial disease. Her diabetes was more difficult to control than that of the typical diabetic, with unexplained lows that would last for hours and unexplained highs that went on for days. Her leg strength and balance were a continual concern. We were even more desperate for a companion to help manage her diabetes and provide her with support—both physical and emotional.

In the summer of 2009 Rachel invited us to attend the very first Wildrose Kennels Diabetic Alert Dog Workshop. We were excited and anxious to be among experts in the field of dogs and diabetes. We travelled to Wildrose for the workshop with our non-alerting collie in tow. We were eager to see if it was our approach to the training that was wrong or if the dog was wrong. We found both to be true. The next set of winged strangers entered our lives—Mike and Cathy Stewart, the owners of Wildrose Kennels. Mike worked with our dog and us to see if it was possible to train in an alert that had never presented itself. He never asked for a penny. He was patient and kind, a true dog whisperer. The sad conclusion was that our dog wasn't fit for diabetes work. For us this was another heartbreak.

During the first conversation that I had with Cathy Stewart tears streamed down my face, as I begged her to help us find a dog for Anna Grace. As tears filled her eyes, she promised that she would do everything she could to help us. Mike also promised that he would help us any way he could. The Stewarts knew that we had depleted all of our funds, plus donations from friends and family members on a dog that hadn't worked out. Still, the Stewarts pledged to help us.

At this first workshop, we encountered a kennel facility that was professional, clean, well-managed, well organized and staffed by compassionate people who did the right thing. We travelled home from the Wildrose workshop and made the hard decision to place our existing DAD as a therapy dog with a local family. She was a sweet dog with great public access skills. She deserved a life filled with lots of people. We all were sad when we placed her. We loved her, but we knew that she would never save Anna Grace's life. We settled in to wait for our Wildrose Kennels Diabetic Alert Dog.

We learned during that next year that the staff of Wildrose doesn't just meet you, sell you a dog, and send you on your way. They learn about your family. They learn about the diabetic. They learn about the journey, the trials, the tribulations, and the pain. They share in the pain that is forever a part of the disease. The Wildrose staff embraced Anna Grace with their love. During our visit to the kennel they treated her like a normal kid and allowed her to meet the puppies and the mama dogs. They allowed

Anna Grace to roam the property and enjoy the freedoms of the beautiful kennel.

We heard from Rachel regularly and started our second effort to raise funds for a DAD. We found it embarrassing to go back to our family and friends and admit that the first dog didn't work and we wanted to try it again. We wanted them to once again dig deep into their pockets and help us provide Anna Grace with her lifesaver. The amazing thing about Wildrose is that it was never about the money. It was never about a magic number that we had to reach for them to talk to us and help us. They committed to helping us on day one without hesitation. Their commitment to us was pure and motivated out of love and hope for Anna Grace. They also recognized that failure was never an option.

After nearly a year of fundraising and waiting, Rachel shared with us that a black Lab puppy had been tagged to become Anna Grace's Diabetic Alert Dog. We were thrilled. Rachel cautioned us that there was much work to do. She cautioned us to be patient. Like all parents waiting for a lifesaver, we were eager and impatient. Anna Grace named the sweet black puppy with eyes filled with wisdom and spirit J.D., for Juvenile Diabetes. Rachel communicated with us constantly and spoke of J.D. with such pride and knowledge. She made sure we knew the good, the bad and the ugly about J.D. He was shaping up, Rachel said, and turning into a great dog, but a very high-energy dog. We heard what Rachel told us, but we didn't always listen. Rachel reported that J.D. had a solid alert to blood sugar fluctuations. He was developing good public access skills and he was very driven and energetic. What could be bad about that? During this time, we received confirmation that Anna Grace did in fact have a mitochondrial disorder that affects the energy production in her body and in every organ. It was heartbreaking to have another diagnosis. We also watched her continue to struggle with her leg strength, her balance, and her coordination. All of these are part of the mitochondrial monster.

We travelled to Wildrose Kennels in the spring and met the beautiful and spirited J.D. He was an amazing dog with a very high energy and drive, as Rachel had said.

The Wildrose staff once again devoted their time to helping us gain confidence and knowledge in managing J.D. They spent endless hours working with us. Wildrose dogs are wise and well trained—it is the would-be owners that need the help. J.D. could alert to Anna Grace's blood sugar fluctuations, but he could also be too much energy for her to handle. Again, in our own ignorance and desire to have Anna Grace's dog, we overlooked the high drive and energy. We convinced ourselves that it could be overcome through time and training.

***

We happily took J.D. home with us against Rachel's advice. She didn't like the match. We worked with him daily for hours in an attempt to build his bond with us, and to develop Anna Grace's ability to control him. Rachel knew she wasn't going to get the popular vote when she told us to send him back, but she knew J.D. wasn't ready for Anna Grace and she knew that Anna Grace wasn't ready for J.D. Through tears and turmoil and worry, we sent J.D. back to Wildrose Kennels. J.D. needed a different diabetic to take care of. Anna Grace needed a different DAD. Once again we were heartbroken. How could we be back here? How could we be without a dog again? Rachel called and checked on us often. She cried with us at the disappointment of another failed bond, but Rachel gave us her word that she would find the right dog for Anna Grace. Mike Stewart also called and made the same pledge.

Months passed and we decided to attend a July workshop with Wildrose in Colorado, its summer location. Rachel told us that there was going to be a dog there that might be able to work well for Anna Grace. She cautioned us to not get our hopes up, but to go with open minds and hearts. We travelled to Colorado and learned more about these amazing animals and the work they can do. We trained on public access work, controlling a dog, learning a dog, and learning to trust ourselves. We were hopeful that we would be leaving with a dog and waited anxiously for Rachel and Mike to decide if we would in fact be paired with a dog.

Through tears, Rachel once again had to tell us that they did not have the right dog for Anna Grace.

Tim and I had just watched Anna Grace's body ravaged by a seizure brought on by a diabetic low the night before this news. We were desperate for help. We felt such despair when we knew that we weren't leaving with a dog. Rachel and Mike had watched Anna Grace all weekend. They studied her mobility and gross motor delays. They knew that sending us away with anything less than perfection would be another failure. So we all tearfully agreed that we would wait on the right dog. We returned home and our days were once again filled with endless doctor's appointments, trying to find the right treatment and help to manage Anna Grace's newest diagnosis. Surgery was scheduled for January 2011 to have a muscle biopsy done to further define her disease and help with a treatment plan. Anna Grace struggled horribly to recover. Her surgical site became infected. Her energy plummeted to a low level that we had never witnessed. She became sick with streptococcus for weeks. Her little body had struggle after struggle after struggle.

On a cold and cloudy January day, Rachel called with a surprise—a dog named Keeper. She was a four-year-old, yellow British Lab with a sweet and gentle spirit. She had a strong alert, but was mild and timid. Rachel made plans to bring Keeper to us in February. We prepared our hearts and our home for Keeper's arrival. Anna Grace had the flu for weeks with a high fever, high blood sugars, and no energy. As we drove to the airport to meet Keeper, we worried about the possibility of another failed attempt. Tears streamed down my face as I watched the sweet, yellow Lab sniff and nudge Anna Grace. Keeper was the perfect size, and gentle. Anna Grace sat down in an airport chair with Keeper placed next to her. Keeper's nose went to the air and she reached over and grabbed the bringsel attached to Anna Grace's belt loop. Keeper alerted to a high blood sugar after only being with Anna Grace for five minutes. I could not believe my eyes. I sat down and watched in awe as the bonding and love flowed between Anna Grace and Keeper. Keeper was true to her name.

Rachel spent many days with us entrenched in training for Anna Grace, Keeper, and our family. She worked patiently with all of us. We travelled to Washington, D.C. We went to restaurants, to doctor appointments, took public transportation, and visited the library. We went everywhere that Anna Grace would go with Keeper. The two of them worked well together. Keeper snuggled in bed each night next to Anna Grace's head with loving eyes. Rachel attended Anna Grace's school and held a presentation for Anna Grace's classmates about service animals and their importance. Rachel educated the students and the staff. We practiced a school fire drill with Keeper. She proved herself steady, dependable, and worthy. More than that, she made Anna Grace feel safe. Slowly, Anna Grace's self-esteem and independence started to return. She began to walk to the end of our very long driveway to go to the mailbox without a parent. Keeper was her parent.

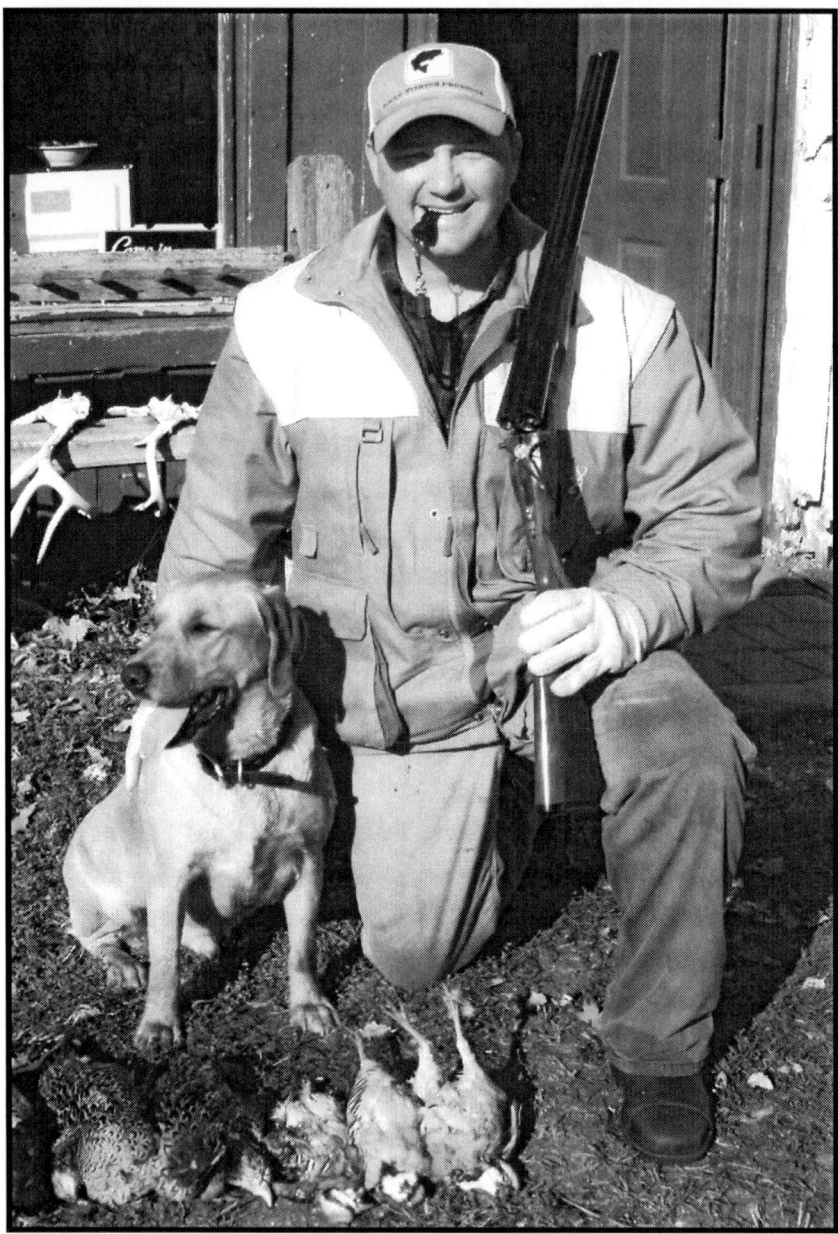

Hatch and Duane V. Miller.

Hatch and Duane V. Miller:
Multitasking

UNTIL THAT VALENTINE'S DAY IN 1990, I had been—or at least I thought I was—a healthy eighteen-year-old athlete. I loved the outdoors, activity, and even competition. But now I was in Mercy Hospital in Miami learning about a disease that was crippling my body. My mood swings, odd appetite, constant urination, and unquenchable thirst started making sense.

Later that year, our family moved from Miami to Colorado for the love of the outdoors. I spent much of the winter on a set of skis. The balance of the year I spent hiking, backpacking, camping, fishing or whatever else I could do in the Colorado high country beneath the blue bird sky days and starlit nights. I was managing my diabetes and felt my energy and attitude restored.

In early 2012, I started noticing a change in my diabetes, which I brought to my physician's attention. I had since moved to Georgia and was running a successful real estate appraisal business and guiding floating fly fishing trips for an outfitter a couple days a week. My blood work was coming back good and I was in overall good health. However, I was noticing that it was becoming increasingly difficult to wake up in the middle of the night when my sugar was low. It was as if I was barely able to make it to the refrigerator for a snack, and once I got there I wanted to eat everything and anything in sight, frantically trying to get my sugar to come up. For anyone who is diabetic or suffers from hypoglycemia, this feeling of helplessness can be very frightening, especially knowing you are at the doorstep of seizure. My physician suggested that we consider an insulin pump, but I decided it did not fit my lifestyle. The insulin pump is fantastic technology, but the idea of being attached to a machine 24/7 never settled with me.

Among my outdoor passions was bird hunting. For several years, I had been researching bird dog breeders, and through an Internet search I found Wildrose Kennels, located in Oxford, Mississippi, best known for its outstanding retrievers. I learned about the "Wildrose Way," a non-aggressive method that uses positive techniques to instill confidence in dogs. The method uses a form of pack leadership to get results. This was music to my ears and I knew I had found the breeder of my next pup. I continued reading and just when I thought it could not get any better, I read about the Diabetic Alert Dog (DAD) Program at Wildrose Kennels.

Already known for their dogs with amazing scenting ability, Wildrose Kennels got its first request for a diabetic alert dog back in 2008. Rachel Thornton informed Mike and Cathy Stewart that she and a friend were using puppies from Wildrose progeny to alert type 1 diabetics to high and low blood sugar. Soon after, Wildrose began the Wildrose Diabetic Alert Dog Foundation and a DAD training program. I contacted Cathy Stewart at Wildrose and she put me in touch with DAD advocate Rachel Thornton, who shared with me that the main use of DADs was to prevent seizures as a result of low blood sugar. I explained to Rachel that my physician was suggesting that I go on an insulin pump and that I was opposed to this. She reassured me that a good DAD would help me with this along with providing companionship, and would serve as a constant reminder to take care of my disease. *Wow,* I thought, *a dog that can travel with me wherever I go that I can train to retrieve upland birds and ducks. A best friend that has excellent manners, doesn't talk too much, and has a dauntless desire to make me happy.*

I began thinking about what I wanted my new dog to be like. I thought back over the character traits of all the dogs I had ever had and chose my favorites from each to develop an outline. First of all, I wanted a male. I also wanted a dog that was loyal, loving, eager to please, amiable, determined, funny, smart, dauntless, easy to train, and determined. And I realized that it was necessary to choose a name for him, so the name game began. As an avid fly fisherman, I turned to this hobby for ideas and came up with the name Hatch, inspired by the time of day when certain bugs hatch from the river and fill the air with swarms of insects. A time when the trout go crazy and gorge themselves on whatever is hatching, lowering their guard and making it easier for the fisherman to catch otherwise elusive fish. I came up with Hatch's full name, "Wildrose Rusty Spinner Hatch," inspired by the rusty spinner fly used in fly fishing, one of my greatest joys in life. And, as a man who refuses to follow the herd, I found a unique name like Hatch a fitting one.

✳✳✳

The time finally arrived to travel to Wildrose Kennels and choose my new best friend—or maybe he would be the one choosing me. I was a bundle of nerves as I flew from Atlanta to Memphis and rented a car to drive the hour and half southeast to Oxford, Mississippi, home of Ole Miss and Wildrose Kennels.

My goal was to attend the orientation, pick Hatch up, and have time to return to Memphis and back to Atlanta all in the same day.

It was a hot day in Mississippi and I was a few minutes late to the start of the orientation. The group was huddled together touring the grounds. Wildrose Kennels is by far the nicest canine breeding and training operation I had ever seen—a business whose owners are in love with what they do and believe in their methods. My attention was immediately drawn to Widgeon, the proud father of my pup. This stud was imported in 2008 from Jonesborough in Northern Ireland. He was trained and had hunted ducks and snipe in the mountains. His superior genetics had made exceptional hunters and diabetic alert dogs. Widgeon's disposition was calm and collected, yet proud and self-assured. Seeing this beautiful Labrador with his fox red color made me hope the tour would soon be over so that I could *be chosen,* as by this time I was convinced I was a mere participant in a master plan orchestrated by divine intelligence.

After meeting Widgeon, I began observing the male puppies that were in a play maze area set up like an obstacle course. It was finally my turn to pick, and the pup I had my eye on from the start came over to me and looked me in the eyes as if to say, "Hello, Duane." This little guy was different from the rest. He was always first through the maze, independent from the influence of the others. I placed him at the start of the maze and he quickly wound his way through to the finish each time to receive his reward. He interacted well with the other pups, jumping right into a tug-of-war, yet he did not need the rest of the litter for entertainment. He was a confident boy with a gentle disposition, yet with a tenacious desire to do what his mind set him to do. I picked him up and he immediately relaxed into my arms. As I held him like a baby, he looked me in the eyes and licked my face. His puppy breath was sweet and fresh. I looked at Cathy and said, "He is the one."

We waited to have photos taken with Hatch's parents as I held him in my arms. During this time, we stood in the sun and Hatch was very unhappy about being hot. When his mother was brought over for the photo, Hatch showed more signs of discontent and an obvious attachment to his mother, which was a great sign for the bond that we were sure to develop in the coming months. The hotter he got, the more vocal he became, barking, crying, and making a scene. The rest of the new owners looked at me as if I had definitely chosen the wrong pup. What they did not know is that Hatch chose me. Hatch's display of attachment to his mother gave me a glimpse into his character, and confirmation of one of the traits I had hoped for. I put his little diabetic alert vest on him and we loaded up in the car and drove off into the sunset, marking the official start to our journey as patient and caregiver.

I decided that a plane ride would be too much for Hatch, so I abandoned my plan to fly, and drove the rental car to the Atlanta airport where my truck was parked. We arrived home late at night and Hatch was beat from the trip. My wife and my nine-year-old son, who were waiting with great anticipation for the new arrival, greeted us. Hatch was immediately introduced to his toys, which he embraced from the start. Hatch waited to relieve himself outside and slept very well at night. He would whimper when he had to go out and I would spring into action to avoid a disappointing situation. At first I would wake a couple of times a night but soon it was once a night and eventually, at about sixteen weeks, he was able to wait until morning as long as I allowed him to go out just before bed.

The toughest part of training for me was learning how to maintain my position as "pack leader" or "alpha wolf." I watched how easily Hatch would move up the totem pole past my wife and son. Every opportunity he got to dominate, he took. I learned from this observation, and as difficult as it was at times, I had to take immediate action when the situation called for it. When "spot training" Hatch, I hated picking him up by the scruff of the neck and calmly returning him to his designated spot. At first he would cry the whole way and my wife would cover her ears. Eventually, he paid close attention to the cause of the correction, and he avoided making those mistakes. I cannot over-emphasize the importance of spot training.

My sponsor at Diabetic Alert Dogs, Rachel Thornton, was available to answer all my questions. I had made the decision long before purchasing Hatch that I would do the training myself. I had trained several dogs in the past and after reviewing the Wildrose Way, I was confident I was up to the task. Looking back, however, I had taken on a very big responsibility and would caution anyone considering a DAD to weigh the options; training is a very big commitment and may be best left to the professionals. But I wanted the pleasure of training Hatch myself and I especially wanted the bond that develops between the dog and his master.

My real estate appraisal firm that covers four states. Our base of operation is Blue Ridge, Georgia, a small rural town close to the state line intersection of Tennessee, North Carolina, and Georgia. I committed to take Hatch everywhere with me and from the moment he got home we focused on basic training. I established and followed a strict routine and Hatch began anticipating my every move. I found that the closer I stuck to the plan, the easier it was to teach him what I expected. At first, the training sessions were short and to the point, following suit with Hatch's short attention span. We made training fun and rewarding and all corrections were non-aggressive yet swift.

Early on, I focused on the basic commands sit, stay, heel and come. We took daily walks on a leash where I taught Hatch how to walk on a lead, and I introduced him to crowds of people so he could gain confidence in a busy and distracting setting. With his vest on, there were very few, if any, places he was not permitted. I read the Americans with Disabilities Act of 1990 (ADA) and was aware of my rights. I also made certain his vest was always on whenever he was working. I noticed after a few months that the moment I placed the vest on him, he interpreted this as "time to work" and responded accordingly, almost as if his attention to me grew stronger.

The toughest part of training was getting my family on board. I had to teach them the proper way to handle Hatch so as not to reverse or contradict any of my methods and expectations. My son, of course, was the biggest violator and Hatch saw Trystin as his littermate and a companion for mischief.

Besides our regimented training, we spent a lot of time exploring in the woods. Every walk was an adventure and early on I taught Hatch the phrase "hunt 'em up." He associated this with finding stuff with his nose and we did a lot of scent type work in order to help him instill confidence in his ability to smell. I would throw a small ball into deep cover, like grass, and send Hatch in after it, always to be rewarded with a treat and "Good dog" upon delivery to my hand.

At the house, I always knew exactly where Hatch was. He never had free run of the house and was always in his kennel or on his spot. I really liked the spot idea because it kept Hatch close by for the low blood sugar work. I made a concentrated effort to take Hatch everywhere with me, including hotels, restaurants, and airplanes. He took his first commercial flight when he was six months old, and has been flying around the world ever since.

We continued bird dog training and at seven months old, Hatch showed his first signs of good breeding from a champion hunter. We were on our way to fly fish at Noontootla Creek Farms in Blue Ridge, Georgia, when Hatch got onto a scent, trailing it to the edge of the brush where he stopped and went into a full point. Curious, I came over to take a look, when Hatch pounced into the cover, flushing out a rooster pheasant. Did I just see what I thought I saw? I signed it off as coincidence, but later, as we were leaving, Hatch went into a full point again, this time flushing out a hen pheasant. I had heard of pointing Labs and was under the impression that this is a trait they either have or do not, one that cannot be trained into them.

By nine months, Hatch was showing the signs of being a "gentleman's gundog." His scent work on the diabetic lows was progressing well, and as expected, Hatch started getting serious about detecting my low sugar. I trained him to alert me whenever my sugar was at 80 or below and he always responded by quietly sitting down in front of me and fixing a dead stare into my eyes. His eyes always get a little bigger when he gets the smell and his nose twitches side to side like the star of the classic television show *I Dream of Jeannie*. If I do not respond, he starts to whimper, and if still no response, he will step up into my lap to get my attention.

***

Up until he was twelve months old, all of Hatch's field training was on bumpers and other types of retriever trainers. The Wildrose Way suggests waiting at least until the pup is a year old to introduce it to real birds. We were invited to a dove shoot in Nashville, Tennessee, so a few weeks prior I started Hatch on a dove stuffed inside a sock. After a few days of this, we transitioned to a dove without the sock so that he could get accustomed to the feel, taste, and smell of an actual bird in his mouth. He had no issues with this at all. He never once tried to chew the bird and successfully delivered the bird to hand each time.

The next task was to get Hatch accustomed to the sound of a muzzle blast. We accomplished this in conjunction with the training with the dove and he quickly associated this with fun, fun, and more fun. With Hatch at a sitting position to my left, my son, standing on top of the truck behind me, would throw the dove out in front of us so that I could fire the shotgun and send Hatch for the retrieve. This worked very well and Hatch more than passed the test in the field as he retrieved close to sixty birds over a two-day period for me and for other hunters. The most impressive aspect of this first hunt was that Hatch was the only dog on the hunt that did not wear a corrective shock collar. Following the Wildrose Way, Hatch successfully retrieved an abundance of birds, each gently delivered. By the end of the hunt, heads were turning and I was a proud papa.

After the Nashville dove hunt, I had a cruise planned to the Mediterranean, and I was torn over whether to take Hatch with me. I decided to send him to Wildrose for a month of advanced training, where they would polish his basic skills and work with him on some more advanced commands. When Hatch was not training, he stayed with Mary, a wonderful trainer at Wildrose who is very involved in the DAD program. Having never been away from Hatch, I worried that Hatch believed I had abandoned him forever. I called Mary every few days just to check up on him and she was sympathetic enough to text me photos. The training proved very successful and Hatch was cared for better than a child.

After the thirty-day boot camp at Wildrose, Hatch and I travelled to Northern Iowa, where we hunted wild pheasant and chucker on a 650-acre farm. It was on this hunt that Hatch developed his pointing skills and showed me he is an all-purpose dog capable of pointing, flushing and retrieving on command.

The fall was chock-full of adventure for Hatch and me as we hunted in Indiana, Tennessee, and Georgia for both wild and pen-raised birds. With each hunt, Hatch's skills became more refined; by late fall, he was hunting like a seasoned veteran. The most impressive skill he displayed was his pointing. He learned to hold the point as long as I wished and we came up with a command for him to wait patiently before flushing the bird. This proved very valuable when positioning myself and other hunters for the flush and shot.

In spite of Hatch being very engaged in the hunt, he never forsook his primary purpose—taking care of me. In Iowa, we were both extremely tired after a day in the field. We had to cover a lot of ground in pursuit of wild birds, and strenuous exercise lowers my sugar more than anything. Hatch woke me up in the middle of the night while I was in the middle of an extreme low. I was close to seizure. I heard him whimpering, but I was so tired that it was difficult to even open my eyes and I fell back to sleep. I woke again to Hatch licking my face and in this moment, I knew I was in trouble. Fortunately I had grape juice next to the bed, and after a few gulps, I had the confidence to go to the refrigerator. After pillaging the kitchen for a few minutes, I rewarded Hatch with a big piece of turkey and thanked him for taking care of me and we returned to get as much sleep as possible before the next day's hunt.

In Indiana, Hatch stopped in the middle of the hunt and sat directly in front of me, looking up at me with what I call his "alert eyes" and he informed me that my sugar was low and it was time to stop for lunch. While I was hunting in Tennessee with my brother, Hatch woke me up in the middle of the night just as my sugar was dropping. I attacked the Fig Newtons with a vengeance. I found out on this trip that Hatch likes Fig Newtons as well.

✳✳✳

Hatch and I start almost every day the same way. At seven, the alarm goes off and while I am in the shower getting ready, Hatch waits patiently on his bed, where he stays all night without fail. Once I am dressed, I call him off his spot and he greets me with the biggest good-morning imaginable, wagging his tail and his whole body in excitement for another day that God has given us. I let him out to the restroom while I prepare our coffee. He comes back from relieving himself immediately and waits patiently at the front door. Highly motivated by food, Hatch is more than willing to do whatever it takes for the mere cup and a quarter of food drenched in salmon oil he gets twice a day. After I prepare his food, he waits patiently, drooling at a sit position until I give him the command "Hatch," allowing him to eat. A few times I have gotten distracted during this routine, returning later to a puddle of drool and Hatch still waiting patiently for permission.

Because I travel for work, there is no telling where the road may lead me. I put close to thirty thousand miles on my truck per year, so one can only imagine how happy I am that Hatch is an excellent traveler. I do not limit where we go, how we get there or where we stay. I always find a way for Hatch and me to be comfortable. I find that with good communication, hotels and airlines are happy to accommodate. I have learned some easy tricks to make our airplane trips very comfortable. I always request bulkhead seating to allow Hatch sufficient room to lie down. Airlines do not charge extra for this special request if they know you are travelling with a service animal. I do not feed or water Hatch on the plane, but I do give him ice to stay hydrated. Most airlines will go the extra mile to accommodate you and I find that everyone is kind, loving and more than willing to help make our trip comfortable.

In addition, I travel with the proper credentials. Hatch has a service dog vest and an official ID that slips into a clear pocket on the side of the vest that displays important information, including his registered service dog number and his DAD number. The back of the card has the phone number to the U.S. Department of Justice and a summary of the laws regarding service dogs. I also have a duplicate of this card that hangs around my neck on a lanyard when I travel for easy reference. One other item I always travel with is Hatch's most recent vet records, showing that his shots are current and the name and number of his vet. I have never had a problem and I have yet to be asked for this information, but it is certainly nice to have just in case.

I prefer that people do not pet Hatch while he is working. Every now and again I may permit a calm child to say hello, but I have taught Hatch that when we are in public and he has his vest on, he is working. One exception is airport security. I always go through the handicap access line because it takes a few extra minutes to get through security with Hatch. I do not allow TSA to remove his vest. Instead, I put our carry-on luggage through the scanner and sit him outside the walk-through scanner. I go first while he waits and once I have cleared, I call him through. Often, the buckles on his vest or his collar will set off the alarm and TSA pats him down, which he loves. I have thought about taking the metal buckles off his vest and equipping him with a collar that has plastic connectors for travel, but for now this process is working just fine and Hatch gets a little loving from TSA. Back at the office, Hatch lies next to me or on his bed throughout the day. If my sugar gets low, he is right beside me staring me down until I do something about it. At first I rewarded every low with a treat. However, it is no longer necessary to reward him every time as he is happy with an old fashioned "Atta boy."

I take Hatch with me wherever I go. Most of my clients know me as Hatch's dad and most often I am asked, "How is Hatch?" before they ask how I am.

One day we may be in a meeting, the next in a class, only to be in the field hunting birds or on a boat chasing fish the next. Hatch has been miles out into the ocean fishing for mahi and tuna and lying next to me in a meeting with investors all in the same week. He is very adaptable and he trusts I will always take care of his needs, and in return he takes care of mine.

Every evening, we lie in bed watching TV or reading with Hatch next to us. He is not permitted to sleep on our bed, but he enjoys every minute he is permitted to spend with us in this sacred place. He divides his love equally between my wife and me, cuddling next to us both, looking up into our eyes as if to say, "I just love you!" I look back at him and I cannot help but believe in the divine intelligence that has brought us together. I will embrace every minute I have with him and I hope I can show him love and affection equal to what he shows me.

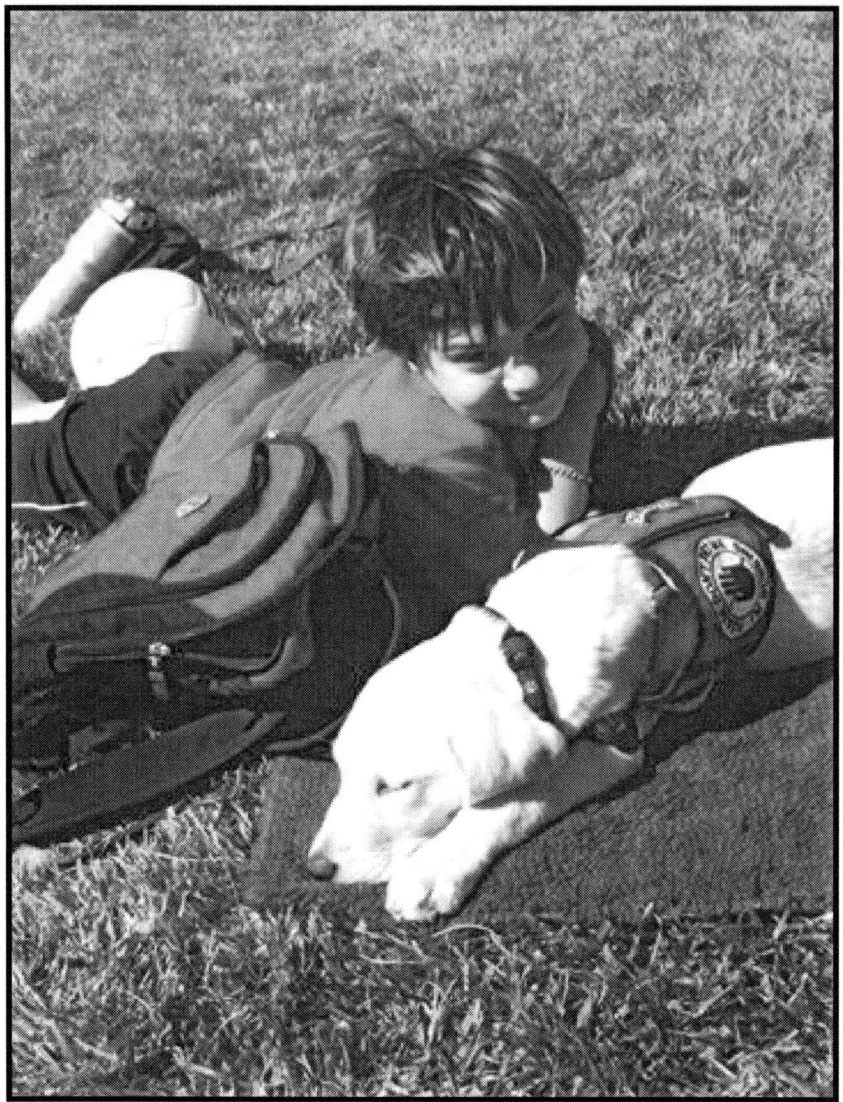

Adam Schwartz and Willow Wonka.

Willow Wonka and Adam and Laurie Schwartz: Redundant Systems

MY ELDERLY FATHER MOVED TO Denver for our family to care for him when Adam was just eight months old. Every day since my father's arrival, we checked "Poppy's" blood sugar, administered insulin, and provided him with daily meals. Adam was an extremely thoughtful child. Each day of his life, my sweet boy had listened to the warnings about the consequences of a poor diet and a lifestyle lacking exercise. He was indoctrinated with the rhetoric that life is a series of choices. He thought choices for a healthy lifestyle would certainly prevent him from a life of finger pokes and insulin injections. How it pains me to this very day to realize how confusing it all was for a young child.

Adam had observed his grandfather's wandering blind right eye from diabetes complications. He had watched how a small scratch on his grandfather's dead-looking diabetic feet could vanish me away from our family for a week to care for him. He had witnessed how a small scratch resulted in a hospital stay requiring intensive antibiotic treatment in the hopes of preventing a toe or foot or leg amputation. Sadly, not all treatments were successful. Poppy did lose a toe, and Adam listened to how we all thought that the outcome was a lucky one.

My heart ached when sweet Adam was diagnosed with Poppy's affliction. In contradiction to everything we had taught Adam about diabetes, his type 1 diabetes was not the result of bad decisions.

"Mom, what did I do wrong?" and "Mom, will I have it forever?"

My heart breaks every time I remember my soft-spoken five-year-old boy looking at me asking only those two very big questions as we drove to the Children's Hospital Emergency Room.

My experience growing up with a parent with poorly controlled type 2 diabetes will forever color the life of my child with type 1.

Unfamiliar with the causes of all the types of diabetes, I attributed all diabetes diagnoses to lifestyle choice, an all-too-common misconception. Diabetes does have a genetic and environmental component. The daily life-long management choices implemented after diagnosis have far-reaching consequences. Our success is not determined by what we must overcome but in how we choose to overcome.

Ignorance about type 1 diabetes is not only in the general population; it is present in the medical community as well. We want to believe that those in the medical profession have all of the answers, and everyone is on the same page, but that is simply not true. My beloved father was a brilliant physician, yet he lived during a time when the understanding of diabetes was rudimentary. He was diagnosed at a time when blood sugar self-monitoring was in its infancy, at a time when nobody recommended strict control over blood sugar levels.

The timing of our son's diagnosis was interwoven with a week-long vacation and less-than-ideal diet choices. It was the last week in May 2008, and our family was taking a vacation to visit my sister in Austin, Texas. From the moment we arrived at the airport, Adam seemed desperately thirsty, making unusually frequent requests for bathroom breaks. The desperation and urgency were eerily familiar. As a child, I had watched my father run to bathrooms in a panic.

As the week progressed, Adam's thirst and frequent bathroom stops remained an underlying issue night and day. Then one night, when Adam took his turn to sleep in my sister's bed, it happened: he wet the bed. This is one of those issues that can easily be dismissed, right? A five-year-old boy wets the bed—is that really a big deal? But it couldn't be dismissed. He hadn't wet the bed since he was eighteen months old. As I helped my sister change the sheets at three o'clock in the morning, I noticed that there was no odor, and the bed looked like a five-gallon bucket had been emptied onto it. There was a copious amount of dilute urine because his body was trying to flush away a chemical imbalance of some type.

My mind raced. To which lecture did I not pay close enough attention? My training as a dentist should have prepared me to identify this condition. I must have missed something. We were given in-depth lectures in all diseases, weren't we? What about my sister, a physician? Shouldn't she be able to diagnosis this awful disease? But neither of us could recall that training when we needed it. What we did have was the familiar feeling that originated from our childhood experience of watching our dad. During those initial moments of my son's illness, there was no medical expertise to come to our rescue, just our life memories.

There is a commonly used expression in medicine when training students to evaluate a patient's signs and symptoms. "When you hear a stampede, look for the horses, not the zebras." Each patient presents with a list of problems, and the student learns how to rule out diseases on their differential diagnosis based on most likely to least likely. My sister and I were trained to look for the common ailments first. Cold and flu are the horses; type 1 diabetes is the zebra.

That night as I crawled back into bed with my husband, I whispered, "I wonder if it is diabetes." My husband whispered back. "Don't look for the zebra. He is five, and he wet the bed—he probably has a bladder infection."

The next day on our vacation, our family outing was a walk around Town Lake Trail. Adam, the youngest of our three kids, is definitely the type not to be left behind. He would be the most likely to run around a lake before ever complaining it was too hot. Yet, there he was, complaining that it was too hot to walk or even to be outside. He had to be carried on my husband's shoulder just to make it back to the car. His feeling of malaise and poor temperature regulation were warning signs that something was really wrong.

That was the last significant incident. The vacation was over, and we returned home. Everything appeared to be normal again: no thirst and no bed wetting for six days. But then it happened once again. We were at a Sunday birthday party, and Adam had a glass of lemonade. That night extreme thirst and a wet bed made their reappearance. Logic would dictate there was no denying that we had a problem. Yet I was still in denial.

So after one more day of denial on my part, I placed a call to the pediatrician's office to set up an appointment. Good, it was handled. We had an appointment scheduled for the next week. But something still felt wrong, really wrong.

Here is a circumstance where many people end up missing their opportunity for an early diagnosis and bypassing a life-threatening crisis. I called the pediatrician's triage nurse and described my concerns, which were thirst, frequent and urgent urination, and unexpected bed-wetting. The nurse's response was, "If he doesn't have any pain or a fever, we will see him next week for his appointment and figure out what is going on."

The next day the nagging feeling, the mother's intuition that something was really wrong weighed heavily upon me.

What else could I possibly check? So the kids all stepped on the scale. Adam had lost five pounds in three weeks! I had weighed everyone before our vacation to get sized for life jackets while kayaking, and Adam was now five pounds lighter. I knew we were in real trouble. No child should lose weight like that with no obvious reason. Adam certainly had not demonstrated a decreased appetite.

I was on a mission to do what I could to answer my own nagging questions. My first task was to get the kids to urinate on a paper stick, Ketostix. That was the easy part. I didn't realize how much fun kids have peeing on something on purpose. But the results made my heart sink. Adam's results were purple, the most abnormal reading possible, whereas everyone else's result was the normal, light tan. Adam's reading indicated the presence of ketones in his urine resulting from a severe imbalance between insulin and sugar metabolism.

Then came the hard part. We used Poppy's spare blood sugar meter on all of us. I made bribes and promises to each child for the finger poke, but they knew, they could tell, I needed them to agree. Each of us had a normal blood sugar reading on the meter below 120 mg/dl, but poor little Adam had two readings of "high." High readings on the meter meant his blood sugar was above 600 mg/dl. Normal blood sugar is between 70-140 mg/dl. I can still recall the gut-wrenching feeling that our lives had changed forever.

After a concerned call to the triage nurse to share our in-home test findings, I received an almost immediate call back from our pediatrician on his day off with the following statement: "Hey Laurie, this is Steve. You need to take Adam to Children's Hospital Emergency Department right away. Adam has type 1 diabetes." That was it—no long differential diagnosis list, no benign options, no discussion of all the innocuous things we would need to try to rule out first. Simply, "He has type 1 diabetes."

I rushed into the bathroom with the door closed to prevent the kids from seeing me fall apart. I needed to be careful and not frighten Adam but I couldn't catch my breath. "Breathe, breathe, breathe…"

Next a call to a family friend, a family practice physician, "Pete, please tell me there is something else."

"No, Laurie, there is nothing else. You need to take Adam to the hospital now."

***

As with most emergency room visits that don't result in hospital admission, there was a lot of sitting and waiting. It took four hours for a blood draw, shot of insulin, and a declaration that we would need to be available for a mandatory appointment the next day. Starting first thing in the morning, during two eight-hour sessions at the Barbara Davis Center for Childhood Diabetes, parents would be taught the basics of how to care for a child with type 1 diabetes.

"You are one of the lucky ones," we were told by the emergency room physician, "Adam can go home tonight because you caught it early." Certainly, "lucky" was not how we were feeling. We were feeling like we had received a severe body blow, and we couldn't catch our breath.

There was no sleep for me that night or many nights since. I believe very strongly that our life journeys are punctuated by the choices of our loved ones. My son's life's journey will be punctuated by my life's choices. I am a dentist not because of an interest in teeth, but because I was a decent math and science student and chose a career path that I hoped would eventually better my future family.

So what did enduring four years of study in dental school teach me, besides how to drill and fill a tooth? It taught me how to find answers, to decipher medical information, and to grasp medical terminology. It taught me how to review the current research in areas with which I was unfamiliar, to study the mechanisms of action of the disease process, to comprehend the properties and interactions of drugs on the patient, and to understand the risks and complications that result from a disease process. It gave me the tools to get "up to speed" on this condition that our family would now face day and night.

That first night on my Internet quest for information, I learned that type 1 diabetic children may go low in their sleep and die even without signs or seizures. I discovered that there is no data being collected to determine what the cause of death was for those lost souls. Even medical examiners typically make a declaration that the cause of death is from complications secondary to type 1 diabetes without understanding the cause. From that night forward, I would not sleep without fear.

Most nights, and sometimes multiple times each night, I would wake to my husband leaving our bed to check Adam with a blood glucose meter. For a long moment, as he moved between rooms, I would hold my breath. I would wait and would wonder about the sound he would make when he reached the kids' room should he discover Adam was gone and quietly cold. I would hold my breath until I heard the reassuring sound of a meter bag being zipped open.

The diabetic research community supports the strategy of tight, aggressive glycemic control, which is essential to prevent long-term complications. If a person with type 1 diabetes can avoid the complications of severe lows (seizures, coma, or sudden death) in the attempt to simulate normal control, then he or she can realistically bypass the complications caused by chronic high blood sugar (including, but not limited to, amputations, blindness, and kidney failure) and live a seemingly normal life span. Prior to the discovery of insulin, type 1 was an agonizing death sentence. The discovery, production, and use of manufactured insulin have prolonged the lives of type 1 diabetics since the early part of the twentieth century. That being said, the use of synthetic insulin, regardless of delivery by injection or pump, is not without risk. In fact, it has very dangerous risks and side effects. Exogenous, or artificial, insulin is not a cure for type 1 diabetes, but an artificial life support system.

Almost everyone, thanks to Hollywood movies, has an image of a person on life support—tubes, drugs, and sudden emergencies. In these dramatic scenarios, we picture occasional dose miscalculations or plugs being pulled and then the patient's impending death. Synthetic insulin is a life support system of the same magnitude, and a person on insulin therapy has a tenuous existence that can be threatened by the failure of the artificial support components at any single moment. Just as a ventilator or bypass machine malfunction can be lethal, a miscalculated dose of an insulin injection can end a life.

What makes synthetically produced insulin so dangerous? It is not natural. It does not behave naturally. Insulin controls the quantity and balance of energy in the blood that keeps our brain alive. Synthetic insulin is slow and long-lasting in its action, which is completely opposite from the insulin that our bodies naturally produce. Once we inject insulin, we cannot remove it. Over the next three to four hours, the state of the person with diabetes could change, causing the dose to be inappropriate. Type 1 diabetes is a condition in which synthetic insulin is not only required for the food consumed, but also for other very important underlying metabolic functions. All of the body's requirements for injected insulin are estimated in dosing. That's right: a powerful, potentially lethal drug is needed every moment of the day and the dosing is nothing more than a guess.

Children get sick, become excited, and have bursts of activity. All of those changes need to be considered in the second-by-second dosing regimens. We see a thirty percent decrease in the total insulin that Adam requires solely based on his level of activity. That decrease of insulin is crucial because he is more sensitive to the effects of insulin with increased activity. But that sensitivity is also dangerous. We have watched the excitement from a new video game cause an extreme high for hours. Those high blood sugars due to a child's excitement result from the release of adrenalin, and require additional insulin to correct. How much additional insulin is needed is an estimate, but we know it will take two to four hours to be effective.

***

There are many more tools available to help manage diabetes, but at many times they give little comfort.

Within two months of our son's diagnosis, we were using a continuous glucose monitor (CGM). The CGM has a small filament that is inserted under the skin. Complex mathematical formulas interpret the information from the sensor and transmitter to predict the blood sugar. In 2008, CGM technology was very new but unreliable. As with many electronic devices, there are imperfections in the system, design, capabilities, and individual components. Batteries need charging, transmitters run down, and plastic parts break. A monitoring system with alarms was better than nothing at all, but because of its failures and hiccups, the CGM was little comfort in the middle of the night.

In March 2010, we were almost two years into life with diabetes. We felt fortunate because we were seemingly doing okay in managing the challenges. Our children were being schooled at home, and we had a home business that afforded us the flexibility to be available for Adam and his diabetes management. Our family had changed over the two years, in many ways for the better. Our previous commitment to a balanced diet was ratcheted up significantly. Exercise was a consistent daily activity, including endurance sports, which improve insulin sensitivity. All three of our children embraced the opportunity to be year-round swimmers on the University of Denver Hilltopper recreation team. Exercise and proper diet became a focus of our entire family. My husband would later say, "Living with diabetes had focused our family like a laser on better health."

Adam's blood sugar control was very good, but not perfect. Our biggest concerns still were the lows that we inadvertently caused and the worry we had that he would crash because of our management choices. We still feared the potential for a low emergency without our constant monitoring. We needed more reliable monitoring options.

***

We began our quest for a diabetic alert dog without fanfare. Our introduction to the diabetic alert dog concept came simply through a chatty conversation I had with my sister in Texas. She was excited to share that she had seen a patient, also with type 1 diabetes, who mentioned diabetic alert dogs. Supposedly, a news report out of Denver had profiled a dog trained to smell blood sugar changes in a child with type 1 diabetes. This little-known type of service dog was being touted as able to ward off health crises through trained alerts.

A few minutes on the Internet to search for local companies led to information that would launch our family into a life-changing journey.

We found www.diabeticalertdog.com, an open information forum run by Rachel Thornton. It was that night that we discovered that Wildrose Kennels was hosting an information conference practically in our back yard.

Wildrose Kennels had an auxiliary kennel facility in Buena Vista, Colorado, and was offering a training conference about diabetic alert dogs. They were offering a training conference for trainers and families alike, simply with the goal of sharing training information.

After a phone call to Wildrose Kennel's co-owner, Cathy Stewart, we were on an alternate course. It was not the path simply to buy a dog, but a quest to become educated about diabetic alert dogs. Our last minute inquiry limited our attendance options. The conference lasted all weekend long: Friday evening and all day Saturday and Sunday. Cathy said, "We are all full, actually overbooked, but some of the attendees are still travelling in and will be absent Friday. Y'all can come on Friday night, meet some other people, and hear what the teams are talking about." That was good enough for us. We decided this opportunity was not to be missed. When Friday arrived, we piled our family of five into the car and committed to drive an hour and a half each way for that three-hour evening conference.

That first evening was mind-blowing as we truly emerged from disappointment and skepticism to a realistic anticipation of the possibilities. We were sitting four feet away from Mr Darcy, Abi Thornton's diabetic alert dog. We observed this adolescent red British Labrador retriever settle professionally next to Abi. Then, thirty or forty minutes into the conference, he lifted his head, flared his nostrils, turned in her direction, and then was up with a happy tail to alert her. Abi, with maturity beyond her years, responded with quiet, calm pleasure to Mr Darcy, checked her blood sugar, and then after confirming the alert, offered him a warm demonstration of gratitude. His task complete and acknowledged, he settled back down quietly at her feet. Watching Mr Darcy alert to Abi, watching young Lilly, also a red British Labrador, alert to her type 1 person Reb, and hearing the real health benefits that were offered by the timing of the alerts amounted to an experience like no other.

That night we heard about night seizures that no longer occurred, because of the dogs. We heard of lows being reversed before symptoms were even noticed, because of the dogs. We heard of dogs that could not only alert the person with diabetes, but would also then run to everyone in the home to get help. Simultaneously, along with these stories were actual alerts, professional and polished alerts as impressive as anyone could imagine. What an amazing experience. What a real opportunity we had, to see, with our own eyes, authentic working dogs. That evening we began to design a mental image, a model of what we would strive to achieve in our own future alert dog.

At the evening's end, with enthusiasm and gratitude, we requested the opportunity to return, if at all possible. Cathy kindly agreed, "Come back, we will make room, yes, join us for the rest of the weekend." So for $150 as the audit fee, our family of five came back for two full days of meals, lectures, demonstrations, and discussions.

Seeing was believing. Observing was beneficial, but the opportunity to walk through town with a service dog was enlightening. Since we did not have a service dog of our own, Mike Stewart provided a dog for our son to handle on the public outings.

***

The foundation of the training for Wildrose Service Companions is calm and focus, and we could see it put into action. Here we witnessed a brief snapshot of the training a puppy receives. We witnessed the foundation of scent training. We delighted in Boss, a little puppy sitting on a cot. Every time our son went low, we were invited to have Adam go over to quietly and calmly be near Boss. Boss would wag his tail, sniff, and Rachel would help him remain calm and focused while he was encouraged to enjoy the mystery odor of a low.

The emotion was raw. We embraced the idea that a dog could smell something that modern medicine has yet to identify and, with proper training, these dogs could prevent seizures, coma and death.

Our amazing weekend submerged in diabetic alert dogs was over. We were physically and emotionally exhausted but tremendously motivated to embark on this adventure. We felt empowered by all the information and direction we had received. We had a path to find additional information and to continue to learn. We were determined to do whatever it took to add this unique monitoring and alarm system into our arsenal of tools for diabetes management. Like many we have met along this journey, once we realized that a dog truly can recognize blood sugar changes and be trained to alert to avert an emergency, we had a sense of urgency to have this dog.

So here we were after completing the Wildrose DAD Conference. We were motivated and ready, but there were no available dogs for sale. Wildrose Kennels was overwhelmed with daily inquiries about alert dogs and had a long waiting list to purchase an untrained eight-week-old puppy. They were closed to accepting new applications for trained diabetic alert dogs. They were not about selling a product. There were no dogs, nor even untrained pups, to be had for possibly six to nine months from Wildrose Kennels. At the Wildrose conference the trainers discussed teaching a service dog self-control by rewarding patience through incremental training challenges based on delays and denials. Delays and denials were not the cornerstones of my educational foundation. "Wildrose Kennels can't be the only game in town to buy a British field bred retriever pup. Why don't you do what you do and get on the Internet, so we can keep moving forward." my husband confidently asked. Call it arrogance or ignorance, but one thing my husband and I don't lack is drive, and we were determined to start without delay. If we failed, it just didn't matter. We loved dogs, and a failure meant our turn on the waiting list would have arrived and we would start over with a Wildrose pup.

Indeed, the lesson was learned. We were now very willing to travel as a family of five wherever required for a possible diabetic alert pup. In hindsight, the terms ignorance and dumb luck come to mind. Within twenty-four hours, we had found a Kansas kennel that had two British Labrador retriever pups available. The kennel was not associated with diabetic alert dog training, but instead focused on breeding dogs for hunting and companionship. All the complexity of training would come later though our efforts. So off we went on a seven-hour drive to get our pup. Everyone piled in the car at five in the morning so we could arrive there at noon, pick up our pup, and set off on our return trip home to be back in bed by ten at night. Our new addition to the family was an eight-week-old yellow female that we would name Willow Wonka. Our seven-hour drive home was wonderful. Our new puppy sat between our boys for the entire trip without fussing or playing or showing carsickness. We were so fortunate… it could have been terrible to be stuck in a car with a new puppy, but it turned out that puppy was quiet, watchful, and a dream come true.

If the dog-training world is small, and the collection of kennels importing British Labradors is smaller, then the diabetic alert dog community is a fish bowl. Everyone knows everyone, and we share a primary goal of helping our children live well with diabetes. What ensued for us was not only a quest to train an alert dog for our son but an odyssey into the humanity of the diabetic alert dog community.

We had studied books on dog training, scent training books, and search and rescue, in addition to reading websites, blogs, and forum posts. We made use of all of these resources. We had learned training concepts at the Wildrose Conference regarding scent, obedience, and public access for a service dog. Mike Stewart's anecdotes about training a hunting dog were absolutely pertinent to living with a dog in the city and guided our training techniques. The images of Mr Darcy alerting and Boss engaging in scent were intertwined with Rachel Thornton's instructions to achieve our goal of a polished alert dog. We pictured the end result, and that helped guide our direction at each step of the journey. We absorbed all details of our observations, every snippet, incorporating them into our goals. At each step, we were intent on finding flaws and failures in our training plan and immediately making improvements.

Got the dog... Ready, set, go. We were doing it and yet we were in doubt. When we watched Willow interact with Adam, we looked for all the ways she was not alerting instead of acknowledging her behavior as recognizing scent. We wanted success, but we wanted it to be undeniable and legitimate. Success would take many months, but what evolved very quickly was a sense of peace and wellbeing.

Those initial days with Willow sleeping in Adam's bed provided the start of peaceful rest for me. We still checked his blood sugar levels multiple times a night, but the frightful unrest and the horrid images of death started to drift away. I wasn't sleeping more hours, but the hours I was sleeping were more restful. I felt that Willow would not stay unperturbed if Adam was having a medical crisis. I felt that at a minimum Willow would not remain still and we would hear her on the room monitor.

What did training progress look like for an eight-week-old, ten-week-old, twelve-week-old pup? Willow did not do all the same things others reported. Willow often responded differently in training scenarios. We placed tremendous pressure on ourselves to succeed, and again, like everything in diabetes, nothing came easy. We were flying solo on this training for our dog, and we had no access to trainers with years of success to guide us. We were silent those first few weeks on the diabetic alert dog Internet forum, and did not make any contact with anyone at Wildrose. We were quiet because we knew we had not demonstrated patience by waiting the six to nine months for a Wildrose pup. But news was out on the Internet grapevine that we had a puppy and we were going it alone on her training.

Then Rachel Thornton revealed her generosity by extending an invitation to us to attend a private training conference at Wildrose Kennels in Mississippi that very next week. We were invited to attend a conference exclusively for Wildrose Kennel clients purchasing and training dogs for hunting and diabetic alert. According to Rachel, that was no problem. According to Rachel, the only thing that mattered was that we were trying to train a dog to help our child live better with diabetes.

Our family of five, with a nine-year-old Maltese and a four-month-old Lab pup packed up for twenty-four hours of driving during the next two days to get to Oxford, Mississippi, from Denver, Colorado.

When we arrived at Wildrose Kennels, it was beautiful. We were physically exhausted from the long days of driving combined with managing diabetes on the road with fast food. I was emotionally uncomfortable and considered myself an intruder, but the Stewarts and the staff were quietly gracious as we entered.

The conference started with an introduction lecture, "Starting Your Pup the Wildrose Way." We were introduced to this information at the previous conference, but now different aspects became our focus. Now those training tips had practical applications for our goals for Willow. We learned to problem solve in our training. Each day that we train, we try to lay a foundation and build on it, and every day we look for problem areas upon which to improve. As we listened to Mike, we gained confidence that we had done well thus far, and Willow was on track.

To my surprise, Rachel confirmed in front of the audience that I had been training with scent samples. She asked me if I thought Willow could find a sample right there, as a demonstration. It was sheer inexperience that led me to reply "Yes." There were approximately two dozen people in rows of chairs and several loose or kenneled dogs. The sample was placed at the front of the room past all of these distractions. Willow had not had exposure to any other dog in two months except Sassy, our five-pound Maltese, and she had never been allowed off-lead in a room full of strangers. Willow had been trained to recognize only Adam's saliva sample during a low on cotton gauze in our home. She had never smelled a sample collected from a different person, she had never been asked to find a sample in public, and she had never been exposed to a sample in a glass jar with a tin lid. There were several factors working against Willow, yet, here I was declaring that Willow, our sixteen-week-old, twenty-pound lab puppy, would find that scent sample.

I hovered at the back of the room, dropped Willow's leash, and asked her to "find." Holding my breath, I watched as she made her way around the room. She sniffed a few people and then moved on. Boy, was I happy that she just sniffed and moved on. She really could have had a field day with the freedom she had been given. She moved to the front of the room closer to the sample, turned back, and then moved forward again. She was in the cone of scent and she was narrowing her search area. Boss, no longer a little puppy, was in a kennel right beside her. She just nosed him and moved right on past to the sample. She located the scent, and she completed her find. Whew! Willow had hit the scent and got the amazing reward of Rachel's sweet voice of praise. That voice of praise elicits joy from dogs, and every dog that I have seen her train responds to her tone of voice with absolute glee.

We felt rejuvenated. It was the perfect time in our training to receive positive feedback, validation and experienced trainer suggestions. Willow demonstrated that she recognized scent, that she could locate the scent, and that she was motivated and persistent. In addition, Willow's focus during obedience work out in the field was good for her age. She was focused on me and was not distracted by her new surroundings. We were ready to continue with our newfound confidence, and we departed Mississippi for our long drive home. Finally, we were participating in the diabetic alert dog community.

In the following months, we would attend four additional training conferences and receive friendship and hours of guidance to navigate the bumps in the road with Willow's training. We were given the tools to be independent, not dependent, in our success. Willow's training centered around fostering her bond with Adam. He fed her, he rewarded, he played with her, and they slept together. Those early efforts to foster that bond has paid off greatly in their relationship. Their bond helped us overcome missteps in training.

***

In the management of type 1 diabetes, a blood glucose meter is used frequently. For us, the meter is used up to twenty times a day. In conjunction with training an alert dog, the meter usage was almost doubled. Each time the young dog appears to become agitated or excited without known cause, it is essential to check blood sugar. Many times during the scent training process, a young pup recognizes the scent and anticipates the reward excitedly. During this stage the alerting behavior is immature and raw but it is important that it be recognized and encouraged. In that instance of excited anticipation the young alert dog is molded to offer a clear signal. But this is also the time in training in which inconsistency in handler response can slow or extinguish the alert training. This was where we struggled.

We later discovered that the glucose meter we were using as the cornerstone of all of Adam's diabetes management and Willow's training was faulty. During the three months after we returned from Wildrose Kennels, Willow provided verifiable alerts. Her alerts were steadily improving in consistency and accuracy. But the following three months were challenging on all fronts. Adam's diabetes management became difficult. It seemed his insulin dosing was always driving highs or lows, but never balancing his blood sugar levels for a moment. His previous state of wellbeing and good control was no longer present. His good nature had evaporated, and his mood swings and fatigue plagued us. Willow's alerts became unreliable and inconsistent. We felt that everything was coming apart, and it was.

Finally, at our quarterly endocrinology appointment, we learned that Adam's blood glucose meter was faulty. The meter, upon which we based everything from insulin dosing to dog training, was inaccurate at least 75% of the time, by a margin of twice that which the FDA finds acceptable. We had lived with and trained by a 40% margin of error. All of those misunderstood alerts were not inaccurate; our precious dog would have to rebuild her trust in us for doubting her.

Dog training depends on communication between the dog and the handler. We had discounted Willow's findings by relying on a faulty meter and failed to reward her for success. Our foundation of consistent and positive reinforcement for recognition and alert of the low scent, so methodically built over six months, had been eroded in three by faulty equipment that caused our inconsistent response to her behaviors.

We were so fortunate that we discovered the faulty equipment and could right our ship. Knowing that we had provided three months of false feedback to Willow's alerts, we stepped back in our training and rebuilt her confidence in alerting. We offered her our best effort in consistent reinforcement, and she responded. She had been reliable all along when the technology was not.

Painful but indispensible lessons are recurrent for us. The experience with a faulty meter drives me to seek redundancy in our monitoring systems. I want backups in place, multiple checks and balances, and I try to focus on context when interpreting information. There is no single device that can present without error. Electronic equipment is far from perfect. Willow filled that technological void. Through Willow's alerts, we are forewarned of shifts in blood sugar. The advanced nature in timing of her alerts provides us with the opportunity to make subtle adjustments in insulin dosing and carbohydrate consumption. The ability to be proactive in medical care instead of reactive in crisis management has meant significant improvement.

Adam's medical tests prior to Willow's arrival indicated that we were achieving near-normal blood sugar averages. Those averages were a combination of time within normal but also a collection of highs and lows. Subsequent to Willow's service we have seen a more realistic approximation of normal sugar. Because of Willow's alerts, Adam not only averages normal blood sugar values, but also maintains a range with fewer fluctuations. Her alerts have decreased, not eliminated, the abnormal values of high and low blood sugar. We witness repeatedly that when she is absent from an activity, our healthy tight range unravels to include more extreme blood sugar readings. Her constant presence is valuable and indispensable in helping us achieve better health for our child.

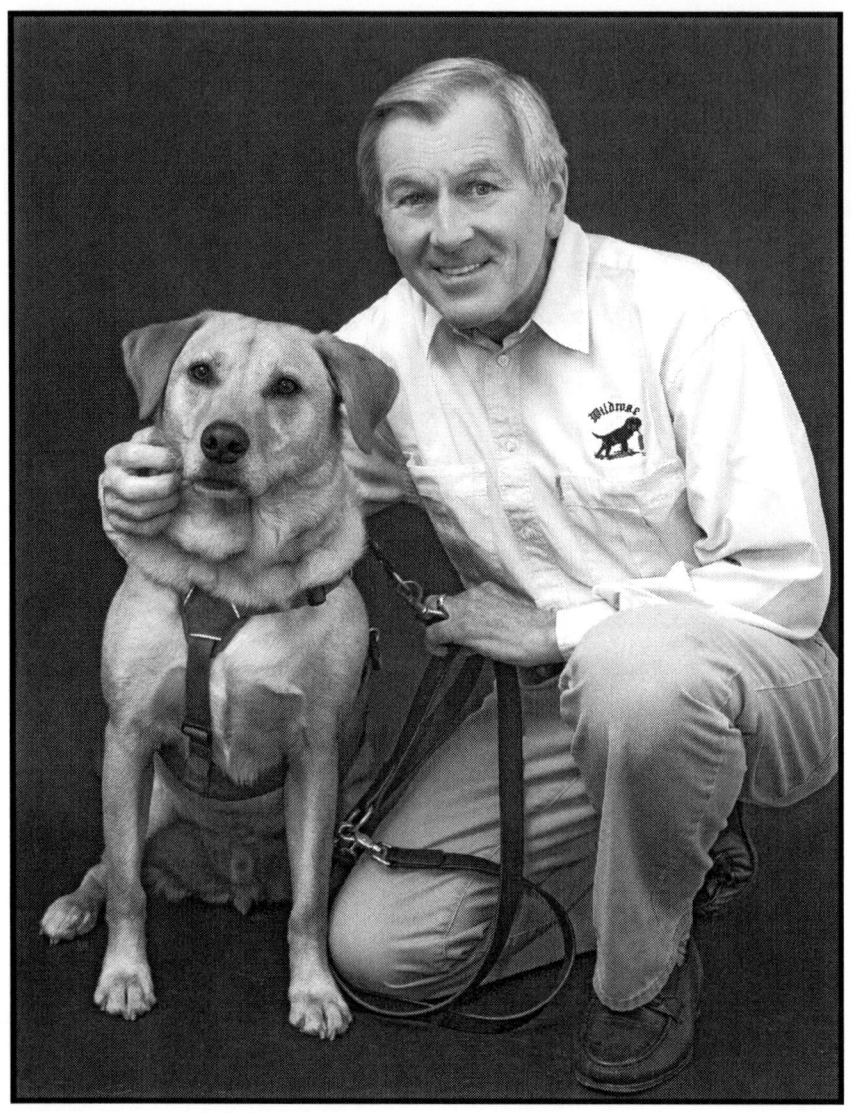

Drake and Tom Arsenault.

Drake and Tom Arsenault with Lisa Mayer: Urban Dog Hero

TYPE 1 DIABETES ENTERED MY life approximately one year after I had been treated for prostate cancer. It's not uncommon for the onset of diabetes to follow a major infection or virus. I was put on oral medications and sent to a nutritionist in an effort to get control of my blood sugars. I'm sure a lot of—or dare I say, *all*—diabetics have been down this bumpy road, some with success. For me, it was a dead end. Frustrated, I found a new doctor and was started on insulin. Finally I had some control over my blood sugar. Life went on with multiple shots daily for years. I got my HBA1 down to 5 and my cancer thankfully stayed in remission into the early 1990s.

The beginning of the new millennium was ushered in and all seemed well. For many years, I was able to feel the changes in my body, which signaled my need for food or insulin. But, in 2005, I started to lose control: rapidly rising and falling blood sugars became a way of life. I became what is known as a "brittle diabetic," characterized by rapid swings in blood sugar levels, accompanied by hypoglycemic unawareness, the inability to sense a dangerous drop in one's own blood sugar. I can, however, remember the first time I suffered its effects. It was Thanksgiving 2006, and I was sitting on my porch talking to my niece, when suddenly, in mid-sentence, I hit the deck unconscious. When I awoke, the porch was filled with firefighters and police officers. An oxygen mask was on my face. Frequently the mask was swapped for a tumbler of orange juice. At one point someone asked me, "Who is the president?" My response was "Johnson," which was accompanied by a shriek from my niece: "Oh, uncle!" Later, after more oxygen and orange juice, I was asked the same question again. My response this time was, "Oh, no. It's worse than I thought…W!" Laughter filled the porch and we went on with Thanksgiving as though nothing had happened.

***

Something had happened, however: the beginning of a different way of life. Calls to 911 to revive me occurred on average every 45 days. I began to know the local firefighters by name. I also became increasingly paranoid, fearful about being alone. Because I couldn't feel the swings in my blood sugar, ordinary chores like shopping and driving were so filled with fear of another episode that I wouldn't do them unless accompanied. The theater, movies, driving—all the ordinary things people do every day—carried new fear, which only exacerbated my condition.

One day, while reading a magazine for diabetics, I happened on an article about diabetic alert dogs (DADs). Finally, I thought, a solution! An online search returned few reputable firms and several warnings of fraud and disappointments. But one site, www.diabeticalertdog.com, recommended the reputable Wildrose Kennels in Oxford, Mississippi. In the spring of 2009, I contacted Wildrose's Cathy Stewart by letter and related my story. She soon telephoned me and when we spoke I could tell she was a woman with an enormous heart. Any doubts I had disappeared.

Cathy put me on a list to receive a DAD from a litter soon to be bred from Turning Teal, or "Widgeon," and Wildrose Brandy. My dog was still a long way away. Not only was he not born yet, but also he still had to be trained. When he was born in September 2009, I got a call from Cathy, announcing the litter had been born. What a happy day. In October 2009, when my puppy, Wildrose Drake, was seven weeks old, he went home with Lisa Mayer, a Wildrose volunteer DAD trainer who had lost her brother to complications from type 1 diabetes in 2008. Lisa trained Drake in the foundations: housebreaking, socialization, place training, obedience, early scent training and public access training. Lisa has trained and competed with dogs in several different disciplines, including her Wildrose-finished dog, Kit. Over the next several months, Lisa and I were in weekly contact via email and telephone. Lisa kept me updated on Drake's progress and sent numerous photos of my hero in training. I described a typical day in my life in New York City to assist her in Drake's training.

The very next day, Drake started going to work with Lisa each day in her law office in Union, Missouri. Her office, on the courthouse square, affords numerous socialization and training opportunities and Drake—ever intelligent and self-confident—quickly became a celebrity around town. He made many visits to the courthouse and other public buildings, and he enjoyed and benefitted from meeting many different types of people in many different situations. Even now, three years later, Lisa reports that people still ask her about Drake and how he is doing.

In November 2009, when Drake was ten weeks of age, Lisa took him back to Wildrose for a diabetic alert dog training conference. It was at that conference that Drake had his first exposure to "low scent" and made his first trip to the Ole Miss campus for public access training. Once he was a little older and his vaccinations were complete, Lisa continued his obedience training with more focus on public access training. By nine weeks of age, Drake was already excelling at "place training" so Lisa used the holiday season as a training opportunity. Drake stayed in place in her kitchen, often for hours at a time, while Lisa was cooking or baking for the holidays. Drake also accompanied Lisa to several holiday parties and family dinners. By the time the holidays were over, Lisa reported that Drake was fully "party-trained." At this time she sent me a favorite picture of him, lying quietly on place on a plaid pillow, staring intently but sweetly into the camera.

Lisa tried to find or create situations that Drake might experience living with me in New York City. For example, because her office is on a courthouse square in a small town, the fire department, police department, and county ambulance are all within blocks of her office. "Each time I would hear a siren, I would put Drake on a lead and take him outside to sit and be steady while the police, fire or ambulance crews drove by. The police and fire crews went out of their way to drive by on training drills, since they knew I was training Drake to become a service dog," Lisa told me. "Drake and I also made numerous trips into St. Louis to ride in elevators in the tallest buildings, walk through crowded streets, shopping centers, and to ride on St. Louis' version of a subway," she said. "Drake impressed everyone he met." When Drake returned to Wildrose, his next trainer told me that he quickly built upon his basic scent training and started "alerting" her type-1 husband within days of arriving in her home.

Finally, in the spring of 2010, I got the call from Cathy to come to Wildrose to meet Drake. She said I should plan to spend a week with them for training, and that, coincidentally, they were soon holding their annual DAD conference, which I might find useful. So there I was, a New Yorker for more than thirty years with a thick Boston accent, heading for the Deep South. I didn't know what to expect. What I found was a welcoming, caring, and generous group of people, intent on making life better for diabetics. If you don't believe a former police chief could fit that description, then you haven't met Mike Stewart, who, together with his wife, Cathy, owns and operates Wildrose Kennels.

I arrived at Wildrose Kennels in Mississippi on Monday, May 3, 2010. The next day, I met Drake for the first time. Before the trainer and I could even exchange a greeting, she told me I should check my sugars because Drake seemed to be "alerting" me. My reading was in the high 200s! Thus began our first week together and the first of many "high" alerts by Drake.

***

One night during that first week in Mississippi, Drake awakened me. I'd forgotten the joy of a dog that needs a walk in the wee hours. When we returned and I settled in again, Drake sat at the edge of the bed staring at me intently and occasionally gave me a gentle nudge. I wondered… Is he alerting? Should I get up and do a finger stick? So I did. My reading was in the low fifties! He woke me up to a low blood sugar! You cannot imagine the incredible joy I felt. Finally, I thought, a solution. I phoned home to spread the joy.

That experience was only the first of many awe-inspiring events at the DAD conference. Drake alerted me during the conference in the midst of a crowd of folks. Outside of Drake, the most extraordinary thing was being with dozens of other diabetics. They come in all sizes, shapes and ages. I'd never had the experience of being with more than one diabetic at a time. It was liberating! I had never felt comfortable doing a finger stick or an injection of insulin in front of anyone other than family. Now, here I was surrounded by people doing just that—or at least some were. Most had insulin pumps, which I had always resisted, thinking it would in some way encumber and restrict my life.

I decided it was time to investigate insulin pumps further

when I returned to New York. In all, it took close to a year to get mine, mostly due to my own reluctance. During that year Drake and I were inseparable. We went everywhere together, and everywhere we went we were educators. People are always curious what Drake's purpose is, and to date I haven't met anyone who has ever heard of a DAD. I like to consider us goodwill ambassadors spreading knowledge of DADs everywhere.

During the time I waited for my insulin pump and since receiving it, Drake has alerted me to high and low blood sugars countless times. Most importantly, he has woken me up close to two dozen times for low blood sugars, which most certainly could have led to diabetic comas and quite possibly death. I had thought with the arrival of my insulin pump, Drake would become redundant, but quite the opposite is true. Countless times, Drake has alerted or woken me up when the continuous glucose monitor showed a safe zone, but a finger stick test would prove Drake correct and the monitor dangerously behind.

In September 2011, Lisa traveled to New York again, this time with the Wildrose pup she was training at the time. Lisa, Drake, WR Missy and I drove upstate to Millbrook, New York to attend the Wildrose retriever workshop at Orvis Sandanona. The first night Lisa and Missy arrived, they stayed with Drake and me at our home on City Island, New York. That night my blood sugar dropped so low that I have no memory of it, but Lisa recollected it this way: "Around three in the morning, I was awakened by Missy whining. I assumed that since she was off her regular schedule because of the airplane travel, that she needed to relieve herself. As I was getting ready to get her outside, I heard Drake moving about in Tom's room and making a few noises. While trying to get her outside, I heard ever-increasing noises coming from Tom's bedroom culminating in a loud crashing noise and Drake's frantic barks. Meanwhile, the puppy didn't need to "air," and she was anxiously trying to get back in the house. Once I heard the loud crash, I knew something was desperately wrong. It turns out that Drake had been trying to rouse Tom for an extended period of time and Tom was unresponsive, so Drake escalated his attempts at waking Tom, and when nothing else worked, Drake jumped up on the bed and literally pushed Tom out of bed onto the floor, finally rousing him. When Tom checked, his meter read 37. When I realized what had happened, and what Drake had done, and that the puppy was whining because she was picking up the low scent, not because she had to tinkle, again, I stood there and cried tears of amazement and joy!"

✳✳✳

Lisa and I became fast friends while Drake was in her care, and we cemented that friendship when we finally met in person. I took Drake home in May 2010 at the conclusion of the Diabetic Alert Dog Training Conference. Lisa and I have stayed in contact and she has made trips to New York City on a number of occasions. Most were training "tune-up" visits, but we manage to work in trips to famous New York landmarks, Broadway shows, and dinners at fabulous New York restaurants. In December 2010, just two weeks before Christmas, Drake and I were walking with friends in midtown Manhattan. Drake had alerted me to a low at my apartment earlier that day. While we made our way through the crowds on the sidewalk in front of the Plaza Hotel, Drake alerted me to another low. It was absolutely amazing. Drake was sitting at heel, calmly and patiently, with enormous crowds swirling around us in the deafening noise that is New York City. Even though I was bundled up in a coat and gloves on a cold, windy December day, he sensed the low. After I treated that low, we continued walking for several more blocks to get to the restaurant for our luncheon reservations. All of a sudden we were surrounded by an unusually large swarm of people. The Christmas Spectacular at Radio City Music Hall had just let out and a couple of thousand people surrounded us. Drake remained at heel, completely nonplussed and steady as a rock. It was then that I dubbed him a "rock star."

***

In 2011 I learned that cancer had re-entered my life. I was diagnosed with lung cancer this time. I was taking a lot of new medications and I was concerned that Drake was not alerting because of the changes to my body chemistry, so Lisa spent a few days with Drake and me in our home, doing some scent work with Drake and teaching me how to "chain" an alert behavior. I recall that she removed some scent samples from the freezer and put them on the counter to thaw. About fifteen minutes later, she went back into the kitchen and opened up one of the samples so she could hide it. Drake was lying on his place on the other side of the house, but within seconds of Lisa's opening the sample, Drake raced into the kitchen and barked. It was apparent that Drake was indeed alerting; I was so relieved.

The social part of our visit was to attend the Westminster Dog Show at Madison Square Garden. Of course, Drake accompanied us to the evening group judging, sitting on his place intently watching each group being judged. Finally, after about an hour, other people in the audience started commenting on Drake's impeccable behavior, likening him to a statue. Drake was still sitting and watching the show intently, not moving a muscle. A few moments later, the non-sporting group came in the ring. Drake was still watching, until the standard poodle in full show regalia pranced around the ring. With that, Drake let out a grunt of disgust and lay down on his place, and didn't watch any of the rest of the show. It was hilarious.

Drake accompanied me to my treatments at Memorial Sloan Kettering Cancer Center (MSKCC) in New York. Although Drake couldn't accompany me during radiation, he was able to be with me during chemo. I think the chemical changes in my body confused Drake's alerting during this time. But, *boy,* did his presence perk up the other patients receiving chemo. The nurses couldn't resist bringing him to visit and elate several depressed patients. By the end of my chemo treatments there was a constant procession of patients coming to visit Drake when we were in residence.

While I was at MSKCC, some of my lung was removed, along with four ribs. A fiberglass mesh replaced the ribs, and two titanium rods were inserted to hold it all in place and allow me to stand upright. But one of the most important results of Drake's and my time at the hospital was enlightening doctors, nurses, and other medical professionals—many who were unfamiliar with diabetic assist dogs—with our amazing story.

I am retired now, and the biggest part of our calendar for the past two years has been our frequent trips into the city for checkups from where we live on City Island. The other big chunk of our calendar has been our twice-weekly class at Port Chester Obedience Training Center. We recently earned our beginner novice title, and soon will be competing in the novice category. I can't recall who it was that suggested we do this, but to whomever it was, I owe a thank-you. Drake enjoys it immensely. He loves using his skills to please me, and he constantly amazes the trainers with his incredibly quick understanding and execution of whatever is expected of him. He amazed everyone one day when he alerted the instructor, a borderline diabetic, when she was having a low!

I recommend joining a training club to anyone with a DAD. As useful, rewarding and invigorating as classes are for Drake, they are equally exhilarating for me. The classes have strengthened the bond between Drake and me and they give Drake some time "off" from his very busy job of keeping watch over me. But it's not all doctors and classes. We go to movies, restaurants, shopping—all the things everyone does in everyday life. Drake has traveled with me on numerous airplane trips as well as on extended car trips. He certainly made a huge impression when I took him to Las Vegas to attend my sister's wedding. We had to walk through the casino in order to get to the room where the wedding was taking place. I heard more than a few exclamations and compliments on the very handsome Drake as we walked through the casino. I guess that's not something people see every day—a perfectly behaved dog walking through a noisy, bustling casino in Las Vegas.

I have been working on this story on and off for the last several months, and had put this writing aside for days now while I pondered what direction to go with it. Nothing had come to me until last night. Drake woke me to low blood sugars not once, but twice! The CGM showed me to be in safe numbers. What more can I say?

***

Drake and I left New York on Sunday, April 28, 2013, starting our drive to Oxford, Mississippi, to attend the annual Wildrose DAD workshop. After traveling for several hours on the interstate, we were about fifty miles from our day's stopping point, when we were sideswiped and pushed into the concrete barrier. There was extensive damage to my car, but thank goodness, no one was seriously injured. When the air bags deployed, including the rear side air bags, Drake was in his usual spot, on the back seat where he can monitor me in the driver's seat. Needless to say, Drake was frightened and unsettled by the accident.

We made our way to a hotel, and rented a car and returned to New York the next day to sort out our nerves, injuries, and the aftermath of the accident. About a week later, still in a rental car, Drake and I went out for the day. We started by going to a movie, followed by an hour-long shopping trip. As we left the shopping center and were walking towards our rental car, Drake started furiously pulling me across the parking lot, away from the car. Each time I approached the car, he physically dragged me away. At first, I thought he was still reacting to the accident a week later, not wanting to get in the car. He was unrelenting in his efforts to stay away and keep me away from the car. After about ten minutes of this, I decided, that perhaps I should check my sugars. I retrieved my meter, and lo and behold, I was below eighty and dropping. Once I treated the low in the passenger seat—the only place Drake would allow me in or around the car—I realized that Drake wasn't trying to stay out of the car himself, but he was sensing my low, and not allowing me to get anywhere near the car, much less the driver's seat. Once my sugar was within normal range, Drake loaded into the car, settled in, and we drove home. Once home, I thought through the events of the day, and realized with tears in my eyes, that Drake had once again saved my life, this time in a very dramatic fashion.

Training Tips for DADs

IN 2012 MIKE STEWART PRESENTED the Wildrose Way in *Sporting Dog and Retriever Training: The Wildrose Way* (New York: Universe Publishing), four chapters of which are devoted to basic dog obedience training. Following these effective methods, a new dog handler can train a pup for purposeful work and steady companionship.

Rachel Thornton developed the methods of scent training and alerting used with Wildrose DADs. Thornton is a mom and nana to type 1 diabetics. She entered this arena with a personal passion for what she knows these dogs can do, having seen powerful benefits for the diabetic and for the family. Thornton has a vendetta against type 1 diabetes, especially against what it does to our children.

The information presented here on scent training and alerting comes from the expertise, which she began developing as she assisted Abi in the training of Mr Darcy. Thus, Thornton is indebted to Mr Darcy, an amazing dog, for what he has done for Abi and for blazing the trail for others in the DAD community. Over the years, other DAD volunteers and trainers have contributed to this pool of shared knowledge.

What can a DAD do?

A well-trained, mature diabetic alert dog is able to alert to changes in blood sugar levels for his partner. DADs offer alerts to fluctuating blood sugar values while their handler is driving, sleeping, working, or playing. DADs are trained to detect low blood sugar, using scent samples from diabetics when the blood sugar value is 75 or lower. The dog must be able to recognize this odor and perform a trained alerting task. The low is believed to be the more subtle scent and also presents an urgent medical need for the diabetic; therefore, training low alerts is the priority.

However, all Wildrose DADs alert to high blood sugar levels as well. While training with a volunteer diabetic, Wildrose dogs are also rewarded for any blood sugar value of 180 or higher. The dogs quickly and eagerly add the high blood sugar (BG) odor to their repertoire. Prolonged high blood sugar levels have dire consequences for the diabetic. The dog's ability to provide proactive information to the handler before high blood sugar levels are at an extreme range is powerful information to the diabetic. By utilizing the information provided by the alert from the DAD, the diabetic can make better blood sugar management decisions. The advanced timing of the alert can help avert a crisis. Or perhaps the alert might interrupt an activity to allow for the reversal of an unexpected diabetic event, such as overdosing for a meal. Undetected pump failure can result in spiking BGs; dogs, on the other hand, are able to alert as the blood sugar values rise, providing the person the opportunity to detect the failure sooner. A diabetic alert dog might also alert to spiking BG, which could be indicative of a forgotten bolus. Many DADs are trained to retrieve the meter or other supplies or even to bring a snack or juice to correct low BG.

Also, getting help from a support person is another very important task DADs learn to perform. Many diabetics experience cloudy thinking skills as their BG drops; in the event that the diabetic is unable to process the information provided by the dog, he should find help.

Moreover, the DADs may well be responding to more than scent. Even though the efficacy of a diabetic alert dog has not been scientifically proven in clinical studies, our diabetics with DADs have plenty of anecdotal evidence. Human bodies are constantly giving off odors through fluids, pores, nose, and mouth. A glycemic event in the blood appears to trigger changes in body chemistry, thus modifying the smells the body gives off—even though no one knows *what* smells the dogs are sniffing. Sure, they smell low BG, but what is a low smell? What exactly is captured in the breath or in the spit or in the sweat of a diabetic during a low event? Nobody knows. No one has found the signature odor, although such research is ongoing. In fact, it is not certain that the work, which the dogs perform, is based one hundred percent on *scent*. As masterful communicators, dogs are astounding discriminators, picking up on cues people don't realize they are sharing. Is there a non-scent component of the DAD's work? How can people train DADs for something of which they have little knowledge? Some mystery surrounds this alerting process. In this section we share what has worked in our experience.

A DAD is not a cure for diabetes. It does not prevent BG changes, but it is able to provide a proactive alert to enable the handler to make medical decisions for better health.

Who can benefit from a DAD?

Type 1 diabetics can find many benefits from a DAD, including improving control over blood sugar level changes. Diabetics prick a finger and check blood sugar level with a meter when they sense low blood sugar; however, diabetics may become hypoglycemic-unaware, unable to recognize any warning signals of dropping blood sugar level. Also, some diabetics struggle with the reliability or discomfort of a CGM (continuous glucose monitor). A well-trained DAD can alert the diabetic when a BG drop is occurring, thus providing extra security for diabetics.

To gain these benefits a person must be able to handle the extra work of managing a DAD, including time for training and the ability to read the dog.

Where did the term "DAD" originate?

Rachel has a vivid memory of when Mike coined the term "DAD." One a sunny day when attendees of the first annual Wildrose Diabetic Alert Dog Workshop trained in small groups around the lawn in front of the Wildrose Trading Company, Stewart was watching Abi and Mr Darcy, who was incredibly focused on Abi. They were doing a few of their "parlor tricks," as Stewart liked to call them. Abi gave no cue to Mr Darcy until he gave her supreme focus. Stewart studied them and then asked someone to take a picture of them: Abi with her braided pony tail and capri pants, bent over slightly, eliciting incredible eye contact from Mr Darcy by holding her finger near her eyes.

Stewart said, "We've got to come up with a name for these dogs. Let's call them DADs." Rachel's husband was slightly offended that Abi might refer to Mr Darcy as her "DAD," and questioned the suggestion. On that hot day in the summer of 2009, Thornton never dreamed that Stewart had coined a term that would not only be affiliated with Wildrose Service Companions, but would also become the acceptable and standard acronym for all Diabetic Alert Dogs.

Diabetic Alert Dogs (DADs) are a relatively new type of service dog. In 2007, when Abi Thornton's search began, there were only a very few organizations training these dogs. The May 2007 edition of Diabetes Health only mentioned three by name. Chat conversations on the Children with Diabetes online forum indicated perhaps two others. There were no open discussions of how these dogs were being trained, no workshops or seminars, and no forums devoted to diabetic alert dog teams—and no Facebook pages.

The familiarity of the Diabetic Alert Dog has exploded in a few years, but it is still a new type of service dog; therefore, it is not uncommon for a DAD team to have many opportunities to educate those around them.

How is a DAD different from other types of service dogs?

One difference lies in the number of tasks the dog performs. The DAD is expected to perform a significant life-improving task: to alert to fluctuating blood sugar values. The DAD might also perform additional helpful tasks such as retrieving a meter or a juice box. However, a DAD may perform more or fewer tasks than other types of service dogs, depending on what is required.

Another difference is that many service dogs have specific times to be on duty or off, which is often distinguished by time "in vest," or wearing the service vest. However, the DAD is expected to perform scent work around the clock, in or out of vest and whether in public or at home.

An additional distinction of the DAD is the olfactory cue to perform a given behavior. There is no verbal cue. Just as the visual cue of an obstruction in the path becomes a cue to the guide dog, an olfactory cue of fluctuating blood sugar becomes the cue for the DAD to alert.

Interestingly, no scientific study proves that there is an odor connected with low blood sugar levels, or that a dog is able to detect it. As mentioned in the introductory chapter, Dr. Dana Hardin, of Eli Lilly and Company, is conducting research into the special scenting abilities of DADs to discover scientific evidence of the volatile organic compounds that dogs may smell emanating from a diabetic's body in, for example, perspiration, breath, and saliva. Empirical data provides ample evidence of the DAD's work. Lower A1cs, tighter glycemic range, fewer spikes and drops, and the resulting confidence for the diabetic are all indications that DADs perform significant scenting tasks that improve the quality and quantity of their handlers' lives. Moreover, some DADs offer alerts at a distance from the diabetic. Depending upon the scent cone and the airflow and a number of other factors, a DAD might alert a third party when the diabetic is not present.

Another distinction is the comparative independence of the person with diabetes. Having a service dog is demanding and draining. The person with diabetes is able to take a break by leaving the dog occasionally, which is not true of many other types of service dog teams. The visually impaired person, for example, rarely chooses to leave the guide dog at home to take a break.

Additionally, a larger percentage of people with diabetes possess the physical and mental ability to train their own service dogs. Many owner-trainers do an excellent job of training to high standards; however, since the owner-trainer is not a professional dog trainer, the finished product might not achieve the same standards as a service dog trained by a trainer with experience, education, and a history in the industry. Nevertheless, handlers must hold high expectations for DADs, not just alerting behaviors, but polished obedience and public access skills as well. To maintain high-level DAD performance and to insure sound public impression, the DAD's behavior must be impeccable at all times.

What does the law say about service dogs?

Anyone with a disability has a right to have a service dog. According to the U. S. Department of Justice, the Americans with Disabilities Act (ADA), defines a service dog as any dog "individually trained to provide assistance to an individual with a disability."

To be considered a service dog, the dog must be trained

to perform tasks directly assisting the disability, which the disabled person cannot perform himself. While service dogs are permitted to accompany disabled owners to any location that any member of the public could go, the dogs themselves have no rights. The access rights belong to the handler; without a disabled handler, a service dog has no rights.

Businesses and organizations that serve the public must allow people with disabilities to bring their service animals into all areas of the facility where customers are normally allowed to go, including restaurants, hotels, taxis and shuttles, grocery and department stores, hospitals and medical offices, theaters, health clubs, parks, and zoos. Business owners of public venues are permitted to ask two specific questions of a service dog handler:

Is this a service dog that is needed due to your disability?
What tasks is the dog trained to perform to assist you?

Various other laws govern the use of service dogs. The Fair Housing Act ensures that applicants or residents of housing be provided with reasonable accommodations; the use of a service animal is reasonable accommodation, even if the landlord has an established policy prohibiting pets. Remember, the service dog is not a pet. Therefore, no additional fees or deposits can be charged for the use of the service dog. Unlike a business owner, however, a landlord can request certain documents from a disabled person.

According to the ADA, the only time a public accommodation is not required to allow a service animal is "when doing so would result in a fundamental alteration to the nature of the business."

Even though the law may sound simple, there are complex matters that service dog handlers need to know, including these:

Each state has state laws.

The Fair Housing Act interprets the law in reference to securing housing with a service dog.

The Department of Transportation, via the Air Carrier

Access Act, establishes the guidelines for air travel.

Title 1, rather than the better-known Title 111, of the ADA gives guidance to employers and employees related to service animals in the workplace.

Bringing a service dog to school can get complex, too.

Service dogs in training (SDiT) are often not covered under the laws governing trained service dogs.

Diabetics with service dogs must educate themselves and cannot expect others to be aware of the laws. As a diabetic with a service dog interacts in the world, he or she must be prepared to be an advocate, a role that involves acquiring a clear understanding of a complex set of laws and being prepared to explain those laws during interactions with people in the world. For further study on this topic, one can consult www.servicedogcentral.com.

Can one receive a tax deduction for using a DAD?

Many medical expenses are tax deductible, and the work of a service dog qualifies as a medical expense. The IRS permits inclusion of the costs of buying, training, and maintaining a service dog as a medical expense. As with any IRS deduction, comprehensive records and receipts are required. Individuals should consult a tax professional for comprehensive advice since tax codes are complex.

What does the general public need to know about service dogs?

Someone that sees a service dog in public should not attempt to interact with it. The diabetic alert dog is working, paying attention to his person's sugar balance. Being in public can be distracting. Adding additional distractions, such as someone trying to engage the dog can delay the dog's ability to provide a timely alert. The dog's focus needs to be on his handler. When people stare, reach out to pet the dog, speak to the dog, throw things at the dog, offer food or make sweet kissy noises, they can cause the dog's focus to leave the handler. This compromises the dog's ability to perform its task. People should ignore the dog the same way they would ignore a wheelchair. Like the wheelchair, the service dog is there to help mitigate some of the effects of a disability. If a people want to interact, they can do so with the person, not the dog.

A service dog usually wears a vest, but not always. The law does not require a vest; however, a handler often puts the vest on a service dogs to make a clear statement to the public that the dog is working. The vest serves as a reminder that the dog is doing an important job and should not be disturbed. In fact, many jurisdictions have enacted legislation that delivers serious penalties to those who interfere with the use of a service dog. For anyone seeing a person with a leashed dog, the best policy is to ignore.

DADs get time off; they are not expected to work 24/7/365; however, since each team is unique, the time off varies. Some DAD handlers join their dog in some type of dog sport that provides the dog the opportunity to be a dog—running, jumping, sniffing, and chasing, for example. We advise our teams to find a hobby that the dog enjoys. Much of what a service dog does is unnatural. The lights and sounds and interactions in public areas are not part of the typical dog's world. Being immersed in the working world can be stressful for a canine. Thus, time off and engaging in a dog hobby can improve the DAD's mental and physical health by providing a release of pressure and tension though play, exercise, or rest.

Even if people cannot discern the task being performed by the service dog, he is working. Some disabilities are not visible to a casual observer. It is inappropriate for people to ask a person why he or she has a service dog or what the medical condition is. Most people do not desire to discuss medical information with strangers. Also, responding to curious questions all day long can be hugely disruptive to the schedule of the DAD team. People need to be considerate when they see a service dog. Just don't ask.

People should not feel sorry for a service dog. Even though there is a good deal of discipline in his life and he has long working days, he is not deprived. He loves what he does. Service dogs are selected and trained for this role because of their potential. They are not overworked; these are working dogs and many would be unhappy not having a working job. Their job provides them with physical, mental, and emotional stimulation.

Where does someone start to learn more about DADs?

Begin by building a base of information about type 1 diabetes, joining a DAD community, and setting goals for your situation.

Your first step is to develop your knowledge about type 1 diabetes. Do this before adding a DAD. In fact, quite a few DAD organizations require a diagnosis of at least twelve months prior to completing an application for a dog. The dog will be capable of providing vital information that the family can only fully understand and act on if they fully understand type 1 diabetes.

Several opportunities exist for joining the ongoing conversations of the DAD community. Social media provide information-sharing opportunities. For example, www.diabeticalertdog.com has a collection of seven years of DAD history. Take advantage of the collection of information that exists on the site's forum. Other unbiased Facebook pages exist to enable teams from many organizations to share information. Consider, for example, the Facebook group "diabetes alert dogs" or the Facebook page "diabeticalertdog.com." Proprietary Facebook pages that exist to promote a specific organization may provide less value in comparison to unbiased information.

To gain insights from experienced DAD handlers, visit with a mature team. Discuss DAD handling issues with the family as a whole and with the diabetic.

Attending a diabetic alert dog workshop allows one to meet with several DAD teams. One can learn a great deal by observing many teams, both novice and mature ones. A workshop also presents work sessions conducted by qualified presenters. And, significantly, the workshop offers a place to connect with other Type 1 families with DADs. These are people to whom you can turn to answer questions and offer encouragement.

Based on the information that you gather, set specific goals for managing diabetes with the assistance of a DAD.

What type of dog serves well as a DAD?

Which dog breeds make ideal candidates for a DAD? Although the breed of dog is not the only aspect to consider, it is an important consideration. A good DAD needs to be:

Adaptable—able to adapt to new situations, people, and environments

Confident—showing no fear around many different types of people, noises, medical devices, and situations

Social/Friendly—able to calmly accept people and other dogs

Focused—not over-friendly, exhibiting single-minded, intense attention to the handler and tasks

Driven—self-motivated to perform the alerting function and serve the handler's needs

Well-mannered—displaying good manners in all situations

Healthy—able to handle stress from working on a slick floor, to remain down for extended periods, and to get in and out of cars

What is an owner-trained versus a program-trained DAD?

Owner training is the process whereby a person with a disability purchases a puppy (at about seven weeks of age), raises, and trains it himself or herself as a service dog. The owner must train the pup in basic obedience, socialization (working in the public), and scenting. With owner training one can get a pup sooner than waiting for a program dog, one that is trained by a professional. Two or three years can be a typical waiting time for a mature, trained DAD. Owner training may be quicker, but not necessarily more effective in the end. There is no guarantee when beginning with a puppy that it will evolve into a good DAD. There is no way to guarantee that the puppy selected will have the proper temperament and nerve strength required to work as a service dog when mature. Sound breeding and adequate temperament testing can help to stack the deck in favor of a working DAD, but it is not a guarantee. Additionally, one cannot be certain that the puppy selected will pass all health assessments at the appropriate age. Finally, any dog can succumb to an injury that delays or ends its work as a DAD. A puppy is a gamble. One can increase the odds, but never be fully confident.

Owner training might also seem appealing because of perceived financial savings. However, this may not be realistic. Well-bred puppies are expensive. Consider these expenses to owner training: a pup from a sound breeding, a breeder who has some type of puppy-enrichment program before the pup leaves his kennel, veterinary visits, supplies, training, and socialization experiences. Over a two-year period, some money might be saved; however, when all funds for training are totaled (including travel expenses to attend training conferences), financial savings may be minimal and should not a compelling factor in deciding to owner-train.

Owner training might be a consideration if one is unable to find an organization with which to work to get a program dog. There are currently a plethora of DAD trainers and more are being added daily. However, the industry is ungoverned and due diligence in selecting one is imperative. (More information on selecting a kennel appears below.) The inability to find an experienced organization with integrity could be a motivating factor in deciding to owner train.

Some select owner training because of the desire to be involved in training one's own dog. For a DAD, this is an especially compelling concept since the dog can begin reinforcement for real-time blood sugar events at an early age. Such puppies might soon begin to show an anticipatory response to the target odor. Additionally, owner training gives one the opportunity to instill specific unique skills that might not be trained by an organization. Flexibility in training compels some to train their own DADs.

Many DAD owners whose first dog was a program dog might consider owner training when a replacement dog becomes a need. Waiting for a significant period of time again for a replacement dog may seem unbearable. Bringing a young pup into the home as the existing service dog matures gives the younger pup the chance to observe and learn from the mature working dog. Not only can the young pup learn by modeling the behavior of the working dog, but after years of being a service dog handler, some handlers feel confident in their acquired skills that prove useful in training the replacement dog.

A program-trained dog, either a young started dog or a more fully trained one, has been trained in the rudiments of DAD work: obedience, socialization, and scenting. The program-trained dog owner continues and maintains the dog's training, beginning with learning to read the dog, establishing communication, and setting a routine. By maintaining close contact with the trainer, the program dog owner can address problems as they arise.

What should one expect in the first few days with a program-trained dog?

Unlike getting a new car, getting a Diabetic Alert Dog (DAD) is taking ownership of a living, breathing, dynamic creature, one with physical, mental, and emotional needs. To build an effective relationship with it, you will need to read your dog, learn to take cues, and take an active, confident leadership role. These are vital to the success of your team. All dogs require a period of transition while they adjust to a new environment and new people. During this period of transition, ask less of the dog. It will need time to adjust to a new handler and new surroundings. Clear your calendar for the first week to make that time as successful as possible.

As you acclimate to each other, you will learn to read the dog and it will learn to respond to the cues of a new handler, one with a different voice tone and different mannerisms from the program trainer. The DAD will have to adjust to the new people, places, and things that are a part of your life. No one should expect a new DAD to alert with perfect accuracy in the daytime, at nighttime, at home or in public. Your consistent training will enable it to become more accurate as you meld as a team. Your program dog is a mature "started dog" that possesses the rudimentary training tools to begin the journey as your DAD. As the owner, you must maintain the dog's training. No training is ever complete. Learning is a lifetime pursuit, both for you and your dog. You will continue to learn together and you will have to maintain all that has already been learned. You will have to address problems as they arise, and maintain close contact with the trainer. Participating in this hard work together will be gratifying for both of you.

How does one select a DAD organization?

Seven years ago, very few organizations offered any diabetic alert dog training. In a few short years, there has been an explosion of organizations providing training and information. The consumer needs to take advantage of this volume of information and spend time acquiring knowledge. Only an educated consumer can make wise decisions.

The diabetic alert dog industry is not regulated. There is no certification process required for DADs. Trainers are not required to possess any credentials. As a result, there are good trainers with poor business ethics and bad trainers who have the best of intentions. The absence of standards or governing authority coupled with the desperation of anxious parents, who fear for the very life of their child, makes this a potentially dangerous industry. To be an informed consumer here are some issues to consider.

Advertising: Is the organization spending a lot of resources self-promoting? Advertising is not needed in this industry. If an organization has a successful team in the field, other diabetics in need will see the working model and make inquiries. Self-promoting in Facebook groups, especially to diabetic support groups, is an undesirable plea to people whose emotions are raw and whose need is great, making it difficult to discern the pros and cons of that advertising.

Cooperation: Does the organization or trainer participate in open online forums like www.diabeticalertdog.com or Facebook groups such as "Diabetes Alert Dogs" or "diabeticalertdog.com?" Proceed with caution if the prospective trainer is not a well-known team player in the DAD community, but rather has formed a closed, exclusive group. Transparency is a desirable trait. There is much to learn from one another and from healthy dialog.

If the online forum has a history feature, use the search engine to retrieve all of the posts from your prospective trainer and ask the following questions:

Does this trainer offer help or ask for help?

Does he or she freely offer help or charge for any help to be provided?

How long has the trainer been involved in online discussions?

What types of questions has the trainer asked you?

Does the timeline you observe in his or her online interactions with clients match the claims made in other areas, such as on the website?

Does the trainer have a relatively recent history but a fast self-promotion to a level of expertise?

If he or she is a relative newcomer, has he or she been prudent in working a few dogs until fully understanding the process? DAD training is complex. Wise trainers begin with a few dogs and see them through to a level of maturity before progressing.

Breeding: If the breeding is not well thought of, with proper credentials and medical clearances, and without adequate guarantee, it could be a most painful journey. Does this trainer breed the dogs he or she places or acquire dogs from an outside breeder? What is the source of the breeding pair and how much experience does this person have in breeding? What types of health guarantees are offered?

Commitment: Training a diabetic alert dog requires long-term commitment. The training process does not end when the dog is placed, but rather moves into a transition period. A young team is not a definitive example of an organization's training success. Has the trainer demonstrated commitment to follow up in order to produce a mature working team? Use caution when the organization's most eager enthusiasts are those still waiting for a dog or those who have had their dog for less than a year.

Training Methodology: Use of aversive devices or force methods is a personal decision but one with which you need to agree. Some such methods have been proven to create fear and mistrust that can erode the core of a service dog. Vacillating between methods creates confusion. Talk to the trainer in order to understand what methods are used and why. Observe his or her mature dogs for confidence in complex environments.

Application Process: Trainers who care are selective not only with their dogs but also with their clients. Since there is a huge demand that can't be met, trainers can afford to be selective with the goal of building a history of success for their organizations.

Additionally, trainers will be selective if they truly care about the best interest of the dog, the diabetic, and the family.

Credible trainers will often have certain restrictions in place with respect to the age and needs of the client or relative to the location of the client. People might initially be offended by those restrictions, but success is more difficult to achieve in a home with very young children or in a home with many dogs or at a location that is a great distance from training support. Restrictions indicate an experienced knowledge of service dogs and their workability, and a strong desire to succeed.

Scent Imprinting: Scent imprinting has its benefits, yet is not the one decisive characteristic of a DAD. Since this is a relatively new technique, the most mature and successful working DADs were never scent-imprinted. It is value added, but it is not particularly resource-intensive for the breeder, so it is not a reason to inflate costs.

Placement Rate: New trainers that start many teams quickly demonstrate a lack of responsibility. Again, DAD training is complex, and wise trainers bring a few dogs to maturity before moving on to others. There are many desperate diabetics seeking help and not enough dogs. Putting a large quantity of young DADs into service makes it extremely difficult for an organization to provide adequate trainer support. Without advanced problem-solving training support and follow-up after placement, the DAD could have a twelve-month window before it becomes nothing more than an overpriced pet.

Trainers: It is preferable to find an organization with stability and therefore consistent training. Here are some questions to consider about the staff of the organization:

How many trainers work with the organization?

How long have they been working for that particular organization and how much experience do they have as trainers in general?

What kind of credentials does each trainer hold?

Do they participate in any type of ongoing continuing education?

What is the rate of turnover among the trainers?

How did the organization become involved with DADs? Is there a keen understanding of the disease with which they are seeking to help? Do they have a personal connection with type 1 diabetes?

Placement of Dogs: Not every dog in training is destined to be a service dog. The area of service dog work with the greatest longevity is the seeing-eye dog and those organizations have learned to expect that a significant percentage of their canine candidates will wash out.

The age of the dog at placement is also a significant consideration. Dogs need to be mature in order to show their nerve strength and their ability to sustain trustworthy transferable obedience skills in diverse environments.

Most reputable trainers do not sell (commit) puppies until about five weeks and they do not let them go home until seven to nine weeks of age. Not every puppy from a litter is destined to be a service dog. While preliminary testing of the litter can give a good indication, it takes months to determine if a pup is capable. Proper testing of puppies reveals that a small percentage is ideal service dog candidates. It is presumptuous to think that each and every pup from any and every litter is qualified in temperament and nerve strength to be a service dog.

Some families opt to accept a young dog as a started dog. To those who are highly motivated to train their own dog and who understand that the dog might fail or fall short, this model might be appropriate. But avoid organizations that sell a pup at the price of a mature dog that has completed developmental milestones. Clients who purchase pups must understand that they are owner trainers in a high-risk venture. If they do not understand that their dollars purchased a pup that has an equal chance of success or failure, then they have been deceived.

It takes time to discern how each pup will mature developmentally in order to match it to a specific person. Reputable service dog organizations have learned that the match between a canine candidate and its partner is a unique and precise fit. A trainer should pay keen attention to the pup and the prospective family and its environment. It is usually best to make this determination after the puppy is twelve months old.

Transparency: Potential DAD clients should seek convincing answers to the following questions:

Can I come to the kennel and training location to observe and meet trainers?

Can I visit a DAD that is currently in training?

Can I examine a copy of the contract prior to any financial commitment?

Honesty and Integrity: Having a DAD is hard work and requires a serious commitment from the prospective client's entire family. A credible organization will be honest about the difficult journey on which the family is considering embarking before taking anyone's money. One can feel trapped when friends and family have donated funds, but the dog isn't working or the process is not working out. An honest trainer will educate potential clients about these issues ahead of time.

When Does Training Begin?

AT FIRST SIGHT YOUR DOG is observing and taking cues from you, so whether or not you know it, you are training your dog as soon as you meet it. Your goal is to train in sound behaviors and avoid dysfunctional activity. To do so, you must begin to read your dog and to establish communication with it. The training process that begins when you first meet and continues throughout your time together involves three facets:

Obedience/tasks
Socialization/public access
Scent work

How does one read a dog and why is it important?
Dogs are excellent communicators. They read people closely and they express their feelings through subtle signals. To read your dog's mood and attitude observe its complex body language, including facial expression (eyes and mouth), ear and tail placement, hair (hackles) and posture. A fearful or nervous dog is in no position to learn, nor is one that is overly aroused or indifferent to your interests. To train effectively and to perform successfully in public you need to know that your dog is in a

sound disposition and a biddable mood. Make adjustments to your schedule as needed to match the dog's emotional needs.

As you live with your DAD, you will carry on a continuous conversation, sharing information and responding to each other. Make your responses clear and prompt. Always be attentive to the dog's subtle signals.

Why is it important to establish eye contact with a dog?

Eye contact between the handler and the dog is an essential act of communication, ensuring that the dog is paying attention to the trainer. The handler establishes eye contact in order to capture and build the dog's visual focus and attention. Whether there is a non-scent component to his work or whether the task is fully scent based, having the dog's focus is a step toward success in all training activities. Getting and holding eye contact with the dog is the first step in giving any command, whether it to find the low, get the meter, or simply to sit.

To establish this behavior with a dog, have it at heel or sitting in front of you. Gain its attention by snapping your fingers or calling its name. When the dog looks at you, return the eye contact steadily and immediately reward the dog, by saying "good dog." With a pup the attention span will be a few short seconds; an older dog can hold the eye contact longer. Work with the dog to sustain longer and longer periods of focus, holding its attention and repeating gently, "good dog." Prior to giving any command, a handler should call the dog's name to capture the dog's attention and then give the command while the dog is focused on the handler.

What basic obedience tasks does a dog need to learn?

The core skills are "sit," "stay," "here," and "heel." Other tasks are also important, including to stay on place, to relieve itself on command, and to leave something alone. See Stewart's book, Sporting Dog and Retriever Training: The Wildrose Way, for more on how to train these skills.

What are some practices that are essential for all training activities?

In order to achieve success a handler should observe some basic practices when training a pup.

Establish eye contact with the pup before giving a command. Remove sunglasses, if wearing them, in order to make eye-to-eye communication. Snap your fingers to get the pup's attention, then say the pup's name and make eye contact. At the beginning expect the pup's attention to be short. Later on, work to extend the period of time that it holds attention and eye contact with you. This is an important bonding activity and it establishes the pup's attention to your communication.

Keep training sessions short at first, just a few minutes at a time, twice a day at most. This will enable the pup to stay focused. When the pup is tired or unfocused, it is not going to learn or perform well and it will dislike training activities.

Never throw a bumper, a ball, or a toy for the pup to run and chase. Only set out retrieves with the dog on a lead and under control. The run-and-chase game will undoubtedly lead to the pup running off with the ball or toy and daring anyone to chase it. Allowing a runaway habit to develop creates a bad behavior that is difficult to break.

Strictly limit the number of retrieves given to a young pup in order not to burn the pup out. Send the pup on two retrieves at most every other day or so.

When the pup reaches four-and-a-half months and begins to lose its baby teeth, cease all retrieving. Pain from sore gums will cause the pup to drop the bumper and to dislike retrieving. Resume retrieving at six months, when the pup's adult teeth come in.

With training activities later in the pup's development, make certain that it can perform an activity five times in five different locations before you move on from one training activity to another. Please make certain that your pup can execute each training activity five times, each in a different location in the house, backyard, park or field, in the water, if that's appropriate. Build the activity into a trustworthy habit through repetition. This is especially important for DADs that will be required to perform in various public settings in addition to the home environment.

To solidify a dog's training performance, introduce what Wildrose trainers call "the stimulus package," which includes increasing the difficulty of an activity and creating distracting conditions. Both of these elements—increasing the complexity and changing environmental conditions—are especially useful in training DADs because they will experience varying situations during outings in public, whether crossing a busy intersection, in a grocery store, a library, or a business office building. See a specific example of complexity in the discussion of scent training below.

How does one instill self-control in a service dog?

Self-control is a priority for service dogs. And, practicing self-control is a lifelong exercise. Look for ways to incorporate ongoing training into your daily life:

Always reward eye contact.

Throughout the day, have your dog wait for your command—when exiting the kennel, exiting the car, and prior to eating.

To build patience and focus into the daily routine of your dog, always have your dog wait at a door for your command to go through it. This training tool could save his life someday, so condition your dog to view open doors as a cue to sit, not a cue to bolt.

Strongly reinforce place training. A raised bed or a folded bed pad is useful in developing place training with a dog when it is still a pup. When the pup gets off place, put it right back on. Whenever it gets off again, place it back on again, encouraging it with the gentle command, "place." The pup will eventually give up, relax, and stay put.

When place training, do not call the pup off place. That is, do not call the pup to leave its place and come to you from the place. That creates unsteadiness when you are around the pup while it is on place. It also encourages the pup to creep off the place when you walk toward or around the pup on its place, resulting in the pup crawling or creeping toward you and scooting off place.

So always walk to the pup on its place, establish eye contact, say its name along with the command "heel," and heel the pup off place at your side. This same principle applies to the "sit" command anywhere that the pup is sitting. If you tell the pup to sit and you walk away from it, do not call the pup to you from a distance. Always go back over to the pup's side, establish eye contact, and say its name with the command "heel," as you walk it off its sitting position.

Why is this important for a DAD to learn good eye contact and to learn to stay on place? Establishing these training fundamentals transfers to the mature dog staying steady in public access work with the diabetic team partner.

Similarly, train your dog to eat only upon command. Tell it, "sit and wait," or "down and wait." Place the food in sight and have the dog hold position quietly. Then, release it to eat with a verbal cue, such as the dog's name.

How does one teach a dog to leave something alone?

"Leave it" is an important behavior for a service dog to learn, as it will come in handy, for example, when the dog is with the handler at a restaurant and crumbs are on the floor. "Leave it" can be used in crowded environments if the dog is interested in sniffing people or items on a shelf. Also, "leave it" could be lifesaving if a pill bottle spilled on the floor, for example.

"Leave it," or a similar cue, means the dog needs to forgo interaction with a particular object or person. It is also useful to redirect the dog's attention to the handler when using this cue.

To teach this behavior, place a few dog food kibbles in your hand and close your fist around it. Hold the hand in front of the dog's mouth. Be still and be patient. The dog will most likely try earnestly to get to the kibble. He might lick or paw or mouth. It doesn't matter. Ignore all that behavior. No need to say anything. No need for eye contact. Use your marker (clicker) to mark the moment your dog disengages. As soon as it makes any movement away from the hand, click and reward with kibble from the other hand. Repeat this step for about two minutes, ending the training session on the dog successfully disengaging.

Resume training, but begin to withhold the click for incrementally longer moments of time. Ultimately, withhold the click until the dog makes eye contact. Continue to train at this level until the dog no longer even attempts to engage. Your dog has now learned the behavior and it is time to slip in the cue or tell the dog the name of this behavior. This time, as you present your hand, say "leave it," click and treat. Repeat for two minutes.

Repeat this process through various other levels of difficulty:
loosely closed fist
open palm (be ready to close if the dog attempts to snatch a bite)
palm lowered toward floor
kibble on floor
dropping kibble onto floor
placing kibble on dog's paws

Each time begin at the very beginning, with a closed fist for higher-valued items like human food. Practice the cue in various controlled settings. Try using the cue while you are in motion. Heel the dog across the kibble placed on the floor.

When the dog has learned that "leave it" means to disengage

and give his attention to the handler, it is ready to put the cue into practice in working settings. Do not try to use the cue before it is solid in the dog's mind. Practice this activity often and reward the dog richly. This is a valuable behavior to a service dog, because it may come upon any number of potentially harmful objects in the home, the store, or on the street. Knowing how to ignore these temptations is vital.

How does one socialize a service dog?

Service dogs are expected to be comfortable and confident amidst a wide range of stimuli. To prepare your puppy for his role as a service dog, it is important to begin the socialization process early and to continue to socialize your puppy in an incremental fashion. Proper puppy socialization involves exposing your puppy to as many new experiences as possible without overwhelming him. Your puppy must be introduced to new people, new places, new animals, car trips, and various sound and visual stimuli.

As in all areas of training, remember to make haste slowly, as Mike is fond of saying. Proceed at a reasonable rate. In the first few months, your puppy will be getting used to you and its new home and family. Since it will not be fully immunized until twelve weeks old, be very careful where you take it. Your puppy should not be exposed to other dogs or the fecal matter of other dogs until it has completed its last round of parvovirus shots at three months of age. Parvovirus is common and life-threatening, causing vomiting and bloody diarrhea that can be lethal for a pup. Prevention is paramount. The virus is present in dog feces, can withstand extreme temperatures, and can live for up to two years in the soil. However, the risk of contracting canine parvovirus should be weighed against the risk of not providing proper socialization to your pup. To completely isolate a puppy until the vaccine series is complete would conflict with the puppy's need for adequate socialization. The critical period of socialization occurs during the first sixteen weeks of the puppy's life. During this time, the puppy needs to learn confidence, basic obedience, and he needs to be exposed to a wide variety of stimuli.

Proper socialization from the earliest age is essential. Things that the pup experiences in the first sixteen weeks cannot be completely erased and will always be a part of who he is; things omitted during this time can never be completely instilled later. All research indicates that from birth to sixteen weeks contains most of the major critical periods in a puppy's development. "After sixteen weeks, the rest of the dog's life is either building on what he learned during that period or overcoming what he didn't." Robert K Anderson, DVM, American College of Veterinary Preventive Medicine and American College of Veterinary Behaviorists states "the risk of a dog dying because of infection with distemper or parvo disease is far less than the much higher risk of a dog dying (euthanasia) because of a behavior problem."

So how do you balance the need for socialization and the need to protect your pup from parvo? Use common sense and limit the puppy's world to safe places, places that are not likely to expose it to parvovirus. Avoid "dog places" such as dog parks, pet stores, and pet potty zones. When you take your pup to the vet, do not put it down on the floor, but hold it in your lap.

Your puppy can become accustomed to touch through grooming and handling of its feet and ears. Invite friends and family over to interact with it. Make sure that it greets them politely by sitting before being greeted. A large percentage of dog training is habit formation. It is never too early to begin building good habits.

During the first three months, you can also expose the puppy to new sounds. Common household noises can be startling to a young pup: blender, dishwasher, washing machine, dryer, pots and pans clattering, hairdryers and, of course, vacuum cleaners.

Introduce these noises in an incremental approach, making sure there is plenty of distance between the noise and your puppy initially. If it is frightened, casually place a little more distance between your puppy and the source of the sound.

During the first twelve weeks, use the rule of twelve, which suggests some of the following experiences for a pup by the time it is twelve weeks old:

Walk on twelve different surfaces (hardwood, concrete, grass, etc.).

Interact with twelve different objects or toys.

Experience twelve different environments (home, car, another house, etc.).

Meet at least twelve new people.

Hear twelve different sounds.

Experience at least twelve moving objects (bike, skateboard, rolling balls, etc.).

Take twelve challenges (stairs, rugged terrain, puzzle toys, etc.).

Eat in twelve different locations or out of different containers.

Be alone at least twelve times per week.

By its fourth month, your puppy is ready to be introduced to the rest of your world. Start slow and small and build on your success. Consider the stimulus value of each encounter. For its first outings, select events and locations that are less threatening. Lowe's and Home Depot are good options for a puppy's first outing. The aisles are wide, the floor is low-threat, and they are typically not very crowded.

An outdoor strip mall is another fun place for a young pup. It is a great place to practice the proper way to greet people and to become acclimated to a variety of people.

Your service dog will need great nerve strength. In other words, your puppy will need to deal with difficult situations without shutting down in panic. Consider the attached list as an incremental approach when exposing your dog to a wide variety of public access experiences. Add any places that you typically encounter in your world.

Four to six months: low-threat locations, such as a home repair store, a park, and a sidewalk

Six to eight months: a ball field, a quiet shopping area, a quiet mall, an office, a book store

Eight to ten months: introduction to "under" in dining settings at an outdoor table or a location with fewer crumbs and food smells, like a coffee shop, a furniture store, and an elevator ride

Ten months and older: grocery store, church, restaurant, and theater

Keep a weekly record of your outings; make a goal to have at least one socialization-training event each day. Note your puppy's strengths and weaknesses so that you can plan for training improvement.

Observe these rules of common courtesy for service dogs in public:

Always clean up after your dog.

Keep your service dog as inconspicuous as possible; when dining, the dog should be under the table.

Permit no sniffing, scratching, or shaking.

Keep your dog clean and well groomed to minimize odor and shedding.

Keep your dog silent—no barking, growling, or moaning.

Wait to introduce a puppy to grocery stores or restaurants until you are confident that it will not sniff or eat crumbs off the floor. Every experience is a training experience. Before you take your dog on an outing, make sure you will be training desirable behavior.

What is an alert?

Every DAD should be trained to give a clear and consistent signal when blood sugar levels are out of range. There are a variety of trained alert signals that can be used, depending on the dog and its handler: nose nudge, paw touch, bow, wave, meter retrieve, and bringsel retrieve. The alert should be clear and distinct but should not disrupt the normal flow of activities in public locations. A vocal alert (barking or whining) is not advised because a dog in public should never be vocal. A vocal dog could frighten someone or disrupt the normal flow of business activities.

How does one select an alert signal?

Nose nudge, paw touch, bow, wave, and stare are among the effective alert actions a dog can make. Do you prefer physical contact or a tattling behavior? Select one that fits the natural abilities of your dog and is easy for both you and the dog. For example, if your dog has a natural oral fixation as a response to the odor and if your dog equates retrieving as reward, then a retrieve-based task is a logical alert. However, if your dog is not a retriever, do not set the dog up for failure by implementing a task that is difficult or unnatural.

So consider shaping a natural response along with weighing the prior history of reinforcement. Retrievers retrieve. Herders herd. They are hard-wired to perform specific tasks routinely. It is a part of who they are, so consider it in selecting the alert behavior.

Does the dog effectively use this behavior at other times to gain attention? Have you rewarded the dog for offering this behavior in conjunction with play or affection? If so, you will find that the dog might quickly revert to using this behavior for an alert signal. Preferably, the alert behavior will be clearly recognizable by not only you but also by others, in the event that you require assistance.

What will this behavior look like as it escalates? Many DADs escalate the alert behavior in the absence of timely acknowledgement. Since a diabetic's cognitive skills are diminished when blood sugar values are out of range, most desire a DAD to escalate an alert behavior until it receives a response. Therefore, think about what your alert will look like as your dog increases its intensity or frequency. Also, imagine how each alert behavior would transfer to various environments and times of day.

Your alert behavior needs to be clear, unique, solid, and consistent:

Clear—The behavior needs to decisively communicate to everyone that the dog is performing a task. It must be unmistakable for you or anyone observing.

Unique—The behavior should be used solely to tell you to check your BG, not to elicit any other response. If the dog engages in this behavior and you reward the behavior routinely, then it will not serve as a unique alert versus a behavior the dog uses to be petted, played with, or aired.

Solid—Some alert signals involve more than one behavior. For example, when a dog gives a nose nudge and then retrieves the meter, it is performing two behaviors, like two links in a chain. In training such a chained activity, teach each one separately until both are solid and strong. Practice each one with the dog in many settings and at various times. Connect or chain the two links together only after the dog solidly understands each one. Otherwise, the dog will likely revert to random, nondescript behavior rather than consistently performing a trained alert.

Consistent—It is preferable to have a single alert behavior for all situations. This is a much simpler scenario for the dog and for you. If one alert behavior cannot transfer readily to many environments, during various levels of activity, then you will need to train a different alert behavior for driving, for jogging, for sleeping, for distance, etc. Choose a single alert behavior and avoid adding complexity to it or changing the behavior from one situation to another.

Here are some common alert behaviors:

Nose Nudge—Physical contact between the dog and the diabetic or caregiver is inherent in this behavior. Many find this a great strength since it is likely to get the attention of a diabetic, even when blood sugar levels have affected his or her thinking skills. There are many variations to this behavior. Either a sustained nose touch or a repetitive nose "punch" is a variation of the nudge. However, there are weaknesses to consider. How would this work as a distance alert? Will this nose nudge be desirable if you are in a business uniform? Is a nose nudge safe while driving? What types of nose nudge variations could you train for driving time?

Paw Touch—Physical contact is also the essence of this effective way to get the attention of the handler. Consider, however, how your dog touches with his paw. Some give a gentle touch, yet other dogs have very rough paw touches that can be painful. Can you shape your dog's touch to be gentle? If you are sleeping and hard to rouse, you might be thankful for the firm paw, but if the paw is so firm that it is harmful, then this is not a safe choice. Likewise, many find it undesirable on rainy days (muddy paws) or when more formally attired for church or workplace. Moreover, this might not be a safe indicator for elderly, very young, or small and frail diabetics, or for any diabetic who experiences lack of balance when blood sugar values are out of range.

Bow—This involves no physical contact, but usually presents a noticeable behavior. Yet this is also a commonly recognized calming signal. Is your dog a nervous dog and does he bow frequently in stressful situations? Select a behavior that is distinct. How proficient is the bow behavior? How much duration? Will the dog hold the bow until you respond? How would this wake you? Can your dog offer this behavior in the car?

Wave—No physical contact, but possibly would escalate to physical contact if not acknowledged. Would you want the dog to continue waving until you respond? If so, then you would need to train the wave behavior to last for a considerable duration. How precise can your dog be with the added duration? Does the wave get lower and lower? Would this alert work well at a distance? Would the height of wave impact how it is recognized? Will this get your attention and that of others?

Stare—Many handlers describe an intense look their DADs give them when blood sugar fluctuations occur. This is beneficial but most likely not a behavior that you would train for an alert signal. It is a quiet, nondescript response. The handler might recognize the uniqueness of the stare, but others probably would not, and the handler might not recognize it if BG was dropping. Many handlers find benefit in teaching their dogs to offer eye contact frequently and to build intense focus from the dog during routine time together, whether training or not. If this is an important concept for you, then the stare would not be a useful tool as an alert signal since it could be readily confused with trained focus. Additionally, unless you are watching the dog, you will miss the stare. How could it serve as an effective alert when you are reading, driving, or engaged in other activities?

Meter Retrieve—This alert behavior is distinct and has practical value since it involves medical equipment associated with your care. Both you and others would recognize it as an alert signal. However, there are a number of factors to consider with this alert behavior. How will the dog deliver the meter to you? Many diabetics tell of their dog dropping the meter on them to wake them if they are asleep. How will you train your dog to bring the meter to your hand on some occasions but to drop it at other times? And how will you help him learn to drop it on you when you are sleeping? Moreover, you must consider where you keep the meter. Is it always accessible to the dog? Is this the indicator behavior with which you would like the dog to alert or is this a cued behavior that you would like to request in response to an alert? Alert behaviors that require another piece of equipment are not desirable for some handlers since it is just something else to keep track of, but presumably you would be keeping track of your meter regardless of the alert signal. Because the meter is a high value piece of medical equipment, teach this skill with a lower-value object first and then transfer it to the meter when the dog masters the task. Train the "get it-hold it-give it" behavior to a high level of proficiency prior to transferring to the meter.

Bringsel Retrieve—This is the preferred alert behavior of a Wildrose Service Companion. We richly reward this trained behavior of holding and retrieving. Hold conditioning begins after all adult teeth have fully erupted and the dog no longer has any pain associated with the process. We want the training to be pleasurable for the dog. We use massage techniques to condition the dog to enjoy holding objects in the mouth calmly and patiently. The training begins with an object that is unfamiliar to the dog and that is only used for this training. We teach cues "hold," for taking an object in mouth with no chewing or mouthing. We teach "give" for releasing an object into the handler's hand. When the dog has learned the behavior and can hold, bring, and give, we transfer these skills to the bringsel. The trainer simultaneously does scent-training exercises. With the dog's eager recognition of the scent and solid understanding of hold, the handler is ready to connect these two events to construct a clear, solid, unique and consistent alert chain with the bringsel.

Vocal Alerts—Barking or whining are discouraged. Any behavior that disrupts normal business activities can result in the dog's removal from that location. Barking in church, a library, a business, a doctor's office, or a theater are just a few of the examples that demonstrate how undesirable this could be. Additionally, it draws undue attention for routine alerts that you can quietly handle without becoming a focal point of those around you.

What is a bringsel and how is it used?

Many dogs are trained to perform an alert behavior by using a bringsel, a short stick or other device that is suspended from the collar of a trained dog, and that the dog takes in his mouth as a signal to the handler that he has located an objective.

It is simply a rectangular piece of fabric, sewed together and stuffed with polyester fiber-fil. Velcro webbing allows the bringsel to be attached to a person's belt loop or displayed in another chosen location. The bringsel is often used in search-and-rescue training to indicate a find. In DAD work, the bringsel might be worn by the handler or kept in a consistent location in the home, car, work, or school.

Bringsels can be chunky or thin, long or short, and are available in a variety of fabrics and colors, even two-toned, which is fun for kids. The webbing can be attached in a breakaway fashion for those dogs that like to actually pull it off and hold it. Alternately, wrap-around webbing secures the bringsel from dropping off as a person moves.

Using a bringsel as an alert signal is not the right choice for all dogs or people. Mr Darcy and many of the Wildrose dogs are trained to alert with a bringsel, because they enjoy retrieving. However, for dogs that are not natural retrievers, the bringsel is not an ideal alert tool. Knowing the dog's abilities and knowing your own preferences enables one to make the best choice for the team. Be true to the dog and yourself without concern for other team preferences.

How does one train a dog for scent work?

In training DADs as Wildrose Service Companions, Rachel and her trainers blend classical and operant conditioning, starting with classical conditioning early by enticing a puppy to sniff an odor and then offering a high-value reward. The dog begins to associate the odor with the high-value reward. When the trainers can see that recognition clearly, they increase the difficulty, by presenting the odor in a different vessel, in a different location, with more distractions. Next, they hide the odor and give the dog an opportunity to recognize and find it.

The trainers also rely on operant or Skinnerian conditioning, a method of learning in which the dog makes an association between a behavior and a consequence. All behavior is a function of its consequences. The process might seem counterintuitive. We think that our words (commands or cues) or signals make our dog do something, or that luring, bribing, or prompting forces the dog to act. However, consequences drive its behavior. Animals do things because they work; they will continue to do what is reinforced. Therefore, the trainers use a behavior chain, a series of behaviors linked together in a continuous sequence by cues and maintained by reinforcement at the end of the chain. Each cue serves as the marker and the reinforcement for the previous behavior—as well as the cue for the next behavior.

Holding the bringsel is one part of that chain. The trainers teach each individual piece or link of the chain as an individual behavior and offer deep history of reward and reinforcement for that specific behavior until the behavior itself is solid. Only then do they connect the links together. A chain is only as strong as its weakest link, so trainers spend time making sure each link is sound.

What are the individual links or components to the chain?

Depending on the end goal, each dog handler can devise the component parts of a chain for the team. Here is a schema of a possible chain:

scent > retrieve bringsel > hold bringsel > deliver bringsel > sit > eye contact > patiently watch BG test > reward

(or) give neutral response if a BG is normal and a recheck, as appropriate. If necessary, heel dog to a testing spot and re-test in ten to fifteen minutes.

Back-chain to link the parts of the chain together by connecting the last piece first, then train the next-to-last with the last, then adding the behavior before that, etc. Back-chaining is most effective. Why? Because the dog is always working towards the most familiar, most rewarded behavior—which has been so richly rewarded that it has become a reward in itself. The behavior at the end of the chain will be the strongest and will reinforce the other pieces.

However, there are so many aspects of training, which take place simultaneously throughout the day. Dogs do a lot of "denials," because self-control and stimulus control are invaluable concepts to a service dog. So hang a bringsel in a visible but out-of-reach location. The dog gets used to seeing it and not interacting with it. Trainers do not want the sight of the bringsel to invite play. The bringsel is not a toy. It is not for chewing, retrieving, fetching—independent of the olfactory cue. Slowly, incrementally, the bringsel will be in more accessible, but controlled, locations throughout the day. Eventually, it hangs from a trainer's waist, on the right side. The dog heels on the left. The swinging and swaying of the bringsel on his heeling side would be too great of an invitation to play. The bringsel is a tool, not a toy. So while training individual behaviors in the chain, the trainers also expose the dog to the bringsel, allowing the dog the opportunity to show stimulus control, self-restraint from going after the bringsel.

Teaching a basic retrieve to the puppy (while it still has its baby teeth) will be helpful when it's time to put the chain together. The dog will already have the concept of delivering items to your hand. When the dog has completed teething, the trainer teaches a formal hold: no chewing, no dropping, only releasing the object to hand on cue. They teach this with a variety of items: a wooden dowel, a bumper, a tennis ball, but not with the bringsel. They do not introduce the bringsel until the dog has learned "take," "hold," and "give" with the other objects. When the dog understands those concepts, the trainers apply those learned concepts to a new object, a bringsel, initially giving a verbal cue. Later the cue fades, replaced with an olfactory cue. While some trainers teach the odor as the original cue, others teach "bringsel" as the cue to indicate that the dog should retrieve and hold the bringsel.

Meanwhile, the trainers have been teaching other behaviors, such as "Where is it?" to locate a person. Eventually, when in the home working for a child, a trainer will want the dog to present the bringsel to the parent, and then lead the parent to the diabetic child, and give the bringsel to receive the reward at the scent source, the child.

How can one save a low scent?

Use a Ziploc brand freezer bag and cotton pads, round or square, available in the cosmetic department of most stores. Make sure they are not scented.

When the diabetic is in a low, but safe range (a BG of 75 or lower), have him or her place a cotton pad in his or her mouth, holding it there only long enough to saturate it with saliva.

Place or spit the pad directly into a freezer bag. Additional scent samples can be made from same low, as long as doing so does not jeopardize the health of the diabetic. All samples from same low can be placed in same freezer bag, but it is helpful if they are not placed on top of one another in the bag, but side by side.

Press all air out of bag and seal it closed.

On the outside of the bag, note the date and the BG number.

Place the bag inside a larger, gallon-size bag. Seal and store.

Store the bag in the freezer in a location removed from smelly foods, such as meat, bell peppers, or onions.

Continue to collect future scent samples for lows, in smaller freezer bags, clearly marked, placing all of them in this larger bag.

When you are ready to use a sample, remove one from the double freezer bag and let it reach room temperature before training with the dog.

After removing a sample from the freezer, do not re-freeze it. Store it in the refrigerator, double bagged, between training sessions. At the end of the third day, discard it.

What type of training should one use to train a DAD?

While there are a number of effective dog training methods, Wildrose trainers use the Wildrose Way as set forth in Stewart's book, Sporting Dog and Retriever Training: The Wildrose Way. Some Wildrose DAD trainers and volunteers supplement the Wildrose Way with clicker training. Rachel Thornton is certified as a Dog Trainer Professional by Karen Pryor's Academy for Animal Training and Behavior, from which emanates the clicker system of teaching that uses positive reinforcement in combination with an event marker. The most common event marker is a clicker, a devise that makes a quick, unique sound. This sound marks a desired behavior in real time and is followed by a motivating reward. The marker is a very precise way to communicate to the dog exactly which action earned the click and its reward. Clicker training is not about using a clicker. In fact, it is possible to clicker train without ever using a clicker; there are plenty of other ways that the trainer can mark the desired behavior. Some common verbal markers are "yes," "good," and "nice."

The difference between using a verbal vs. clicker is that the verbal bridge must be processed by the dog's cortex (the processing part of the brain) while the click is processed by the amygdala (the reactive part of the brain that causes a reflexive action, such as startling when a pan is dropped). Basically, the click causes the dog to react first, then process the action it was performing while the verbal marker must be processed through the cortex before the dog can think about the behavior it was exhibiting. Additionally, the verbal bridge might be less clear to the dog if it is also used in everyday speech; if your bridge is a verbal "yes," you might also use that bridge during conversation with another person. Your marker will be more effective to your dog if it is not used at other times. Additionally, verbal markers can be uttered in a variety of tones: true consistency in tone while you are training is difficult. The click is the same every time it is heard. The key is that the marker must be used correctly and consistently along with the other principles of clicker training.

Training your dog involves three steps:
- Get the behavior.
- Mark the behavior.
- Reinforce (reward) the behavior.

Desirable behavior must be marked first and then rewarded. The marker lets the dog know that it has done the right thing. It is a clear form of communication and is then coupled with positive reward. The marker is a way to bridge the gap between the desired behavior and the reward; it will distinctly mark the desired behavior before the dog ceases the behavior. Mark the behavior immediately, then deliver the reward.

The timing of the marker (click) is crucial; click during the desired behavior, not afterwards. The click ends the behavior and is followed by a reward. Reach for the treat after you click so that you aren't bribing or luring the dog. Always treat if you click. You can treat without a click, but never click without a treat. Click only once.

Always remember that rewards must always be earned—no freebies. The dog must work before being rewarded in order to reinforce a strong work ethic. Much of dog training is habit formation. Seek to capture success, reward success, and build a habit out of successful patterns. Routine and structure and setting your dog up for success are vital to this training methodology. Let your dog anticipate structure and order in your home. Wake early enough to invest time with your dog. One cannot sleep in and then expect to throw a leash on the dog and run out the door to work or school; this will result in training and obedience issues in public.

Wake up; take the dog out to air. Then, offer food and water. Exercise with the dog: biking, jogging, heel work, focus. Give the dog a chance to air again before entering any building. Always think ahead to set your dog up for success. Begin to view the world through the eyes of your DAD.

When you begin training, clear the area of all distractions. The initial learning experience for the dog should be in an environment that facilitates focus. You will add distractions and distance and duration after the dog has learned the behavior.

How does one teach a new behavior?

There are four primary ways to teach a behavior to a dog: capturing, shaping, luring, or manipulating/modeling.

Capturing a behavior: It is simple to capture a behavior if it is one in which the dog naturally engages. The handler simply has to wait for the dog to offer the behavior, then he can mark the behavior and reward it. For example, "sit" is a behavior that all dogs will naturally offer eventually. The handler can wait for the dog to "sit," mark the behavior and then reward it.

Luring a behavior: The handler uses a treat to guide the dog into a desired behavior so that the behavior can be rewarded. The dog's body follows the nose and the nose follows the treat. "Down" is often lured by placing a treat on the ground and waiting for the dog's body to follow the treat to the ground and drop "down." Luring is easy, but also easily "abused;" the dog begins to expect the treat to be part of the picture… as if it is a bribe. Additionally, because the dog is simply following his nose, he is not necessarily thinking. The best DADs are thinking, problem-solving dogs. Luring can be used to produce a behavior but the lure must be faded quickly.

Shaping a behavior: The handler rewards small steps toward the goal, slowly raising criteria along the way. The initial reward is not for the desired behavior but for incremental moves in the direction of the desired behavior. Imagine a staircase leading to the goal; each step up the staircase is part of the shaping plan. Shaping is perhaps a more difficult training tool but is very powerful. Shaping requires the handler to understand the dog's body language and to have good timing. Shaping is a thinking process. The dog learns a lesson and the lesson is remembered.

Manipulating (or modeling) a behavior: The handler physically places the dog into position (pulling up on the collar or lead and pushing down on its bottom to make him sit). This is the weakest training option. It is the slowest and least effective way to train since the dog is being physically forced into position. It requires no engagement or thought process by the dog. It is always best to get the dog to freely offer a behavior rather than forcing the behavior.

A trainer or handler's objective is to change behavior in the dog. However, none of us can truly control a dog's behavior. We can, however, control the probability of future behavior in the dog by manipulating those things which come before the behavior (antecedents) and those things which come after the behavior (consequences). The most fundamental law of training is the consequences determine behavior. A dog will repeat a behavior that is rewarded; that is the basic law of all dog training. There is an illusion that antecedents make behavior happen (trainer says "sit," and then dog "sits"). However, if the consequences of that behavior are unpleasant, the dog is not likely to offer the behavior, even if the trainer/handler gives the cue. The trainer/handler ought to be very attentive to the consequences, considering what is most likely to motivate the dog.

What are some health considerations for a service dog?

Familiarizing yourself with adequate health and nutrition practices for a DAD is important, because health and nutrition will play a big role in your dog's ability to perform obedience tasks and/or scent detection. Learn basic first aid procedures and preventive care, including routine veterinary visits, vaccinations, flea and tick prevention, and parasite control. The following information will help dog handlers care for their DADs.

Health Laws: If you travel out of state or out of the country, research and adhere to the health laws in each area en route as well as your destination. Keep a copy of your dog's health records with you while traveling.

Household Dangers: Be aware of household dangers, such as poisonous plants, chemicals, medications, items that can be chewed and/or swallowed. Keep potentially harmful items out of your dog's reach and do not leave the dog unattended unless it is crated.

Illness and Injuries: Recognizing symptoms of illness, injuries, or nutritional needs is essential in the care and safety of the DAD. Report to a licensed veterinarian deep cuts, lacerations, swelling of any kind, vomiting, diarrhea, loose stools for long periods, ingestion of a foreign body or potentially harmful fluids, rash, dilated pupils, eye injuries, debris in the eye, potentially harmful fluids in the eyes, potential heatstroke or exhaustion, and internal temperature decrease or increase. Keep a fully stocked first-aid kit accessible for emergency use.

Parasites, Both Internal and External: Internal parasites include Giardia (found in stagnant water) and various types of worms. Minimize the risk of infestation by not allowing the dog to drink from unknown water sources, eat anything from the ground, or come into contact with carcasses. Regardless of your attempts to prevent infestation, your dog may be exposed at some point, so deworm it regularly and visit your veterinarian for excessive vomiting and/or diarrhea as these can be symptoms of internal parasites.

External parasites include fleas, ticks, mites, lice, and wolf worms. There are topical and internal treatments to aid in the prevention of fleas and ticks. Research different options and choose the product that is right for you. Some forms of mites and lice can be passed on to humans and other pets; therefore, have a veterinarian treat the dog and other pets.

On the first of each month Wildrose DADs are treated with applications of Heartgard (for heartworm prevention) and Frontline (for flea and tick prevention).

Nail Trimming: Trim the dog's nails and clean its ears as necessary. The nails should just barely touch the floor when it walks. If a dog's nails become too long, it will interfere with the way it walks and can cause serious damage. Walking can become awkward or even painful. Untrimmed nails can split, causing bleeding and pain. Longer nails are more susceptible to being torn, which is not only painful but can also result in infection. So trim your dog's nails twice per month. If you do not trim the dog's nails regularly, the quick will continue to grow along with the nail. When the nail becomes long, the quick become long as well. The quick is the living part of the nail, containing blood vessels and nerves throughout. Cutting into the quick during trimming can be very painful and may result in significant bleeding.

Grooming: Keep your dog well brushed and groomed to reduce shedding. You should give the dog a thorough brushing at least once weekly, but it is a good idea to brush daily to minimize the shedding. A rubber "Zoom Groom" brush is a useful tool for a wet or dry coat. It is a super brush for use during bath time since it is waterproof. When the dog is dry, Zoom Groom collects hair like a magnet that can be easily wiped off. The "shedding blade" can be used like a regular brush when the coat is dry. It will gently and effectively remove loose hair from a shedding dog. The Furminator is another super grooming tool, although more expensive.

Do not bathe the dog more than once per month to prevent the removal of vital oils in the coat. In between baths, you can wipe your dog down with dog bath wipes. These are a quick way to make the coat shiny, remove dirt, loose hair, and foul odors. It is convenient to keep wipes handy to wipe your dog's muddy paws before entering a store or your home.

Dental Care: Because there is a direct correlation between gum health and scenting ability, consult a veterinarian for an ongoing dental care plan. To prevent tartar build up, Wildrose DADs' teeth have been scraped monthly while in training. Poor gum and tooth health will have a direct impact on the dog's scenting ability, because some scent glands are located inside the dog's mouth. Brush your dog's teeth on a regular basis.

Weight: Continuously monitor the dog's body weight. An overweight dog will not perform to capacity and obesity will be harmful to the dog's health. Obesity is the leading nutritional disease affecting dogs in our country. Overweight dogs have greater health risks, including increased joint, circulatory, respiratory and skin problems. A recent survey reported that approximately 50% of dogs in America are overweight. Maintaining the dog's ideal body weight will result in a longer, healthier life and better performance. You should be able to feel the outline of the ribs on your dog; they should not be too easily seen nor should they be difficult to feel. When looking at your dog from above, you should see a clearly defined waist. Proper nutrition for various stages of life involves calorie adjustments to match activity level as well as balancing activity choices for safe growth and development. Consult a veterinarian if you need assistance in managing the dog's nutrition and weight.

Vehicles: If a dog is riding unrestrained in a car, it can be injured by a simple slam on the brakes or a sudden turn. The dog should be in a crate or buckled in at all times while riding in a vehicle.

Exercise and Nutrition: The following discussion of canine fitness comes from an article that Stewart posted on the Wildrose website.

Historically the Wildrose market serviced individual wingshooters, largely people with a background in game dogs. Fortunately for the sport, this is no longer true today. Many of our clients own their first dog for hunting, adventure, and now DADs. Since these individuals have had little experience in the proper care and training of sporting dogs, issues sometimes arise with both health care, conditioning, and even training that would not have surfaced a decade ago. One such topic that needs to be addressed is weight control, nutrition, and proper exercise for the dog. This issue cuts across all disciplines from hunter to DADs. Here are some recommendations:

In the young dog under two years of age, extreme care must be taken to protect skeletal structure. Allan J. Lepine, in his recent study, stated, "It is well documented that the incidence of skeletal disease, including osteochondroses, hypertrophic osteodystrophy and hip dysplasia is markedly increased in the growing large breed dog if management practices are such that this maximal rate of growth is realized… three predominant factors—the dietary concentrations of protein, energy, and calcium are most often indicted." The findings are that hips, knees and shoulder problems that occur in large breeding canines are as much a problem of nutrition and excessive weight as it is genetics. See Lepine's complete study in "Nutrition and Care of the Sporting Dog," published by Eukanuba.

We do not want to promote excessive growth and the dog becoming overweight. Use feed specifically formulated for rapidly growing canines. The protein/fat content must be below 26/16, and likely 24/14 for most large breed canines that do not get the work to burn excessive calories which is commonly the case with our clients. Our Sportsman's Pride puppy feed has now been specially blended for this purpose. Excessively high protein and fat content combined with high calcium phosphorous ratios promote rapid growth, which is harmful to the dog's skeletal structure. Calcium/phosphorous should not exceed 1 % in your puppy feed or adult feed. Use a high quality, highly digestible, balanced food source.

Weight control: The overweight dog is at a higher risk of health issues from respiratory, heart, and even skeletal structure. In many cases the young dog's frame is simply carrying too much weight, which can result in joint problems. Again, pay particular attention the diet and provide a reasonable, low-impact exercise program.

Exercise: Hunters and adventurers, pay particular attention as this is an area that is commonly violated. Keep your exercises with a large-breed dog to low impact and short in duration. Running a dog that is younger than eighteen months for forty-five minutes twice a day under is irresponsible. So, too, is running a year-old dog four miles every morning or attempting to correct an overweight dog by excessively running the dog alongside a golf cart, an ATV, or a treadmill. An overweight dog engaged in high impact exercise may well develop joint problems. Keep exercises short in duration, make them repetitive, involve lots of swimming, and, of course, walking on soft surfaces, such as grass. DAD owners, think about the wear you are causing on your dog daily: slick floors, climbing steps, and jumping in and out of vehicles. Combine this with excessive exercise in duration/high impact, improper nutrition, and not maintaining the proper weight. Disaster awaits. Adventure dog owners: running your dog with mountain bikes, jogging on hard trails, jumping from boulders at too early of an age will result in the same health issues.

Owning a service dog is hard work. A potential owner needs to consider a number of factors: *affording the cost, attending to the dog's physical and emotional needs, giving the dog* downtime, building a relationship with the dog, maintaining training consistency, accepting unsolicited attention, testing your blood sugar more often, and *realizing that the dog may not provide nighttime alerting.*

Affording the cost: Obtaining and maintaining a service dog is costly. Beyond the purchase price, the estimated yearly cost of caring for your service dog is approximately $1,750 including the following goods and services:

Dog food—$50 per month

Veterinary care—$1,000 per year

Equipment replacement—$150 per year

Attending to the dog's physical and emotional needs: Daily consider its needs for food, water, exercise, training, safety, emotional wellbeing, and temperature (including on hot pavement). A DAD is a needy creature. Consider that it will need to be fed, groomed, and vetted. When it gets wet, you will need dry it off. It will need to relieve itself, and you will be responsible for cleaning it up. Whether it is hot or cold or whether it is raining, sleeting, or snowing, your dog will need to go outside to potty. This will happen at times when you may not feel well, at times when you would like to sleep a little later, or at times when it is just plain inconvenient. Adding a service dog to the family is like adding another child. For the child, it is like becoming a parent prematurely. A service dog pees, poops, sheds, drools, throws up, and may even bark, jump, or develop an undesirable habit from time to time. The dog's needs must be tended to like those of a young toddler who is developmentally unable to do many things for himself—it is like having a perpetual two-year-old whom you must feed, water, clean up after, exercise, watch constantly, and reward and correct in a timely manner. A DAD will need this care, especially being rewarded for alerting, even when you are sick and your blood sugar is out of range and you want to be left alone.

Giving the dog downtime: Like you, your dog cannot work

24/7/365. You must discipline yourself and your dog to have a planned time of separation—for him to rest, for you to get a break, and to prevent both of you from becoming dysfunctionally co-dependent. Without planned separation as part of your training schedule, your dog (and perhaps you yourself) will suffer separation anxieties. Since there will inevitably be moments of separation in your lives, prepare for those moments by training for them as you would train for any other event. Plan downtime for your dog by crating it in a variety of places and times of day. The crate should be a place where the dog is off-duty. Make it a refuge for the dog, an enjoyable place solely for rest. From time to time, offer a treat to your dog while it is crated. Occasionally give it a consumable chew stick, and it will associate this surprise treat with crate time.

Building a relationship with the dog: No matter how much training your DAD has had, the two of you will reach your full potential only after you have established a relationship. This central aspect of all that you do together cannot be bought or quickly earned. Consistent communication over time will be the key to becoming the best team you can be.

Maintaining training consistency: You will need to continue training with your dog on a daily basis. Realizing that the dog will never be fully trained nor be perfect, you will need to continue obedience and scent training on a daily basis to continually improve. Dogs can get tired, overly excited, fearful, anxious, and stressed. You, the handler, must be capable of reading the dog and assisting it by managing the stimuli to which it is exposed. Above all, you will need to be consistent, as consistency is a core component of any dog training methodology.

Accepting unsolicited attention: Wherever you and the dog go, you will need to accept unsolicited attention. Someone with a service dog stands out. People want to give dogs lots of attention, even when it is unwanted. At times a business owner or a clerk will tell you that you have to leave because "dogs are not allowed." So you will have to educate yourself about the rights of a disabled person to have a service dog. And you will need to explain those rights to members of the community. You will have to defend your rights firmly but politely. And, you will have to take time to interact with well-meaning, but interfering, people who will not hesitate to stop you to ask about your dog. A normal trip to Wal-Mart will no longer be quick and normal. People will stop you to ask about the dog, to talk to you about diabetes, or to tell you about their dog. Dogs are conversation starters, especially service dogs.

As a diabetic, you have the ability to run an errand or enjoy your typical daily routine without publicly identifying yourself as a diabetic. Some people refer to diabetes as an "invisible disability." Especially with today's medical technology—smaller pumps and meters—your medical condition is not readily evident to the general population during most of your interactions. That changes when you have a service dog. Everyone notices that. They stare. They try to guess (openly) about the nature of the disability or whether the dog is still in training (since they can't identify the need for the dog). It can be frustrating, humiliating, and stressful. You cannot prevent the stares. You cannot avoid the whispers and pointing. If you determine that life with a service dog is the right choice for you, you will need to commit to respectful, responsible dialog with the public, in spite of how they chose to interact with you.

Testing your blood sugar more often: Initially, for months and months as the two of you work to become a DAD team, you will have to check your BG more often, not less, as you learn to read the dog and as you reward its alerting and re-alerting. Since the timing of your reward to a dog is a crucial part of its training, you should always have your meter with you. When the dog alerts, you should check out blood sugar immediately. Not having your meter with you at all times could mean a significant delay between the dog's alert and the BG check to determine how you respond to that alert. You might need to re-check in fifteen minutes. This also adds to costs, because most insurance companies limit the amount of test strips that they will fund. So you may find that you will test more than what is covered by your insurance.

Realizing that the dog may not provide nighttime alerting: Some DADs learn to provide nighttime alerts; some do not. A diabetic who gets a new DAD must realize that nighttime alerting is not automatic. It should never be considered a given or assumed to be a task that a dog can perform consistently. Anyone that wants a dog to alert at night will have to conduct training at night, thus getting less sleep during the process. Several members of our community have testified that they cherish the security that nighttime alerts afford them. However, the reality is that some dogs may never alert and no dog will always alert at night.

In conclusion, having a DAD involves more: more cost, more work, more responsibility, more attention, more finger sticking, and more sleepless hours—especially at the beginning of the dog-person relationship. Everyone in our community that has a DAD knows the great benefits of the relationship, but anyone who is looking to begin must weigh these factors in order to have realistic expectations.

Can one train a dog to work for a child?

Yes, sometimes a service dog is transferred to a partner who requires assistance in handling the dog. The service dog, its partner, and the third party handler are known as a triad team. The parent wisely understands that a young child is incapable of being solely responsible for a service dog at all times.

The DAD working for a child will need to learn to alert to multiple people and often must be capable of being handled by multiple people as well—mom, dad, older sibling, teacher or childcare provider. Each team member will need to understand the cues and behaviors and expectations to continue training in consistency. The dog needs to be capable of interacting with, alerting to, and accepting rewards from each of these people.

The team along with their trainer should fairly assess the appropriate responsibilities for the child and make plans for the support person to assist in the balance of duties. The child should be as involved as possible in the training and management of the DAD; however, ultimately it is the parent who will be responsible to ensure that all health, nutritional, training and exercise needs are rightly addressed.

The child could certainly be expected to feed the dog, offer treats, interact with the dog with toys or balls (as permitted), and offer the high value reward following an alert. The parent or responsible support person will need to provide supervision to ensure safety, consistency in handling, and to ensure that bad habits are neither being encouraged nor reinforced.

Finding a balance between assisting the child and being 100% responsible is important. The child needs to desire to work with the dog, and follow through with that desire in age-appropriate ways.

Are DADs reliable for night alert? What can one do to help a dog make progress in night alerting?

DADs can offer an added layer of protection at night, but no one should ever entrust their health or the health of their loved one to any dog, no matter how amazing that dog is. Any number of factors can affect the dog's ability to alert or can affect the ability of the diabetic to respond to the alert. You should not expect that the dog should accurately and reliably alert on all nights. You should hope for and train for alerts that are an addition to your current management plan.

No one can guarantee a night time alert! Your trainer can condition your dog to a high level of response to the target odor or your trainer might be able to condition your dog to lighter sleep cycles or to anticipating finding a low BG in a bedtime setting but, there is no way to guarantee night time alerting because there are too many variables outside the reach of your trainer.

A strong desire for life-saving night time alerts is the primary reason that many people desire to get a DAD. Carefully guard your expectations in this area. Your frustration and disappointment can be a detriment to your dog's overall success.

In my mind, nighttime alerts represent the most difficult aspect of a very difficult type of service dog work. Work on developing consistent, solid, accurate, reliable daytime alerting and expect that they should precede night alerts. In the meantime, there are a few things you can do to encourage night time alerting:

Train in the bed with scent samples on the diabetic, preferably when his blood sugar is dropping but still in a 'safe low' range. Never put your health in jeopardy in order to train a dog. Train in the bed at any time of day. If you catch a real low, hide in the bed and let your dog search for you, following your low scent. Your dog needs to understand that the alert behavior still happens when you are in bed. In fact, you need to demonstrate to your dog that this is the most valued task he could ever perform for you. Demonstrate this to your dog by making it a lot of fun and using highest value rewards. Dogs do not generalize well, so if you fail to teach him that scent-work and alert behavior happens in the bedroom, in the bed, then he might miss that concept.

At any point during the day, when your dog is settling and just beginning to relax, do some scent training. Not only does your dog need to understand that he needs to alert in lots of different kinds of places (like your bed) but he also needs to understand that alerting must interrupt lots of different activities (like playing or eating or sleeping). You can incrementally increase the difficulty level of this training opportunity by waiting until deeper stages of sleep before placing the sample in front of her nose or increase the difficulty by adding distance (not putting it as close to her nose), but remember to only increase one difficulty factor at time and to make all other factors more simple when raising a criterion in one area. So if you have progressed to the point of having her wake from a deep sleep with the scent directly in front of her nose, add some distance to the placement of the sample, but introduce it at the earliest moment of her relaxing. Slowly build back up to presentation of sample during deeper stages of sleep, with the sample at a farther distance.

Experiment with various positions: both yours and the dogs. Perhaps your dog loves to sleep in bed, yet is not alerting. Move him. Try him in a different spot. Maybe he will be slightly less comfortable and therefore sleep a little lighter if he is on a cot next to the bed. Maybe you have a habit of pulling the covers over your head. You might need to adjust that habit to make this problem simpler for your dog. Maybe your bed is directly under an air vent that is blowing the scent away from you and your dog. Experiment to discern the most likely scenario for success for you and your dog.

Train in the bed using the highest-value reward—even if that is not necessarily the most convenient thing for you. Perhaps your dog's highest value reward is a retrieve down your hallway or a quick game of tug. Consequences drive behavior. Establish amazingly wonderful consequences to encourage nighttime alerting from your dog.

Remember that your dog is a living thing; he responds to stimulus all day long and each day is different. The ability for him to alert at night (or not alert at night) can be attributed partly to his breeding, partly to his training, and partly to your continued diligence, but also greatly to the level of stimulus in his day. On a day when he has been active and alerting, he might sleep harder. On a day that has had additional stress, he might not respond quickly. On a day that he is not feeling well, he might need the extra rest. Your days and sleep cycles are also variable.

Does training need to continue with a program dog?
Yes. Training never stops. Expect to continue training sessions with your dog for the rest of your time together. Training maintains behaviors, sharpens behaviors, and builds fun and helpful new behaviors. Training doesn't need to be an all-day event. In fact, studies show that dogs learn more and retain it longer if training sessions a brief and scattered throughout the day.

Use commercial time during a favorite TV show to do some quick training. Set aside a few minutes in mid-morning to bust up the day and refocus your dog. When you stop at a red light, practice eye contact or name recognition or targeting. Training your service dog is resource-intensive, but you don't have to use large chunks of time nor go to a special class every day.

Donna Hill has a fabulous collection of training videos that are free on YouTube and are organized and indexed for easy access: www.dogvideoindex.blogspot.com/. Use resources like this to teach your dog new skills or refine old ones.

What are some supplies I might need?

Mats
The Gaiam Reversible Travel Yoga Mat is a very lightweight mat, is easy to carry, and can fit in a very small bag, so it makes a perfect travel mat. It provides a clean area for dog to sleep when out in public, without too much bulk to carry. The back side of the mat is a non-stick surface to prevent it from sliding around under the dog. One mat can be cut in half to make 2 "dog places" each weighing 1/2 pound.
www.gaiam.com
Mutt Mats are thicker than the yoga mat, but comes in fun

color combinations and sizes. Each also has a great carrying strap that makes over-the-shoulder carrying very convenient. Durable, nice thickness for dog who isn't fond of cold, hard floors. Wash and dry in machine.

www.muttmats.com/products.html

The Cash Cushion is constructed with one no-skid, wax canvas side and the other side of double sided fleece with a high denier nylon border... rolls and closes with Velcro straps for ease of transport. 29 X 37. Well made. Machine-washable, but hang to dry.

The Mountain Bachelor Pad is similar to the Cash Cushion and made by Ruffwear. It also has one no-skid side and one softer side for dog comfort.

www.ruffwear.com

With either of these, if the dog is wet and muddy, flipping the mat to let the dog lay on the no-skid side allows you to simply wipe the mat with a wet wipe and avoid washing or having a soggy mat.

The four-way—a unique design. Folds flat rather than rolls. Folds to various sizes. Thicker and stiffer than the roll-up types. Very sturdy. When completely unfolded is 36 X 21. Stays closed with Velcro strap.

www.wildrosetradingcompany.com

Leashes

Beautiful handcrafted leather twist leashes. Can be custom made as simple or as complex as desired. Select your own weight and type of leather—even a nice assortment of colors. Fully twisted leash is simple, pretty, and soft. The service is fabulous—both courteous and quick. Very affordable. Will add snaps to both ends and floating rings for service dog, cross-body leash.

www.onlead.biz

Simple affordable hands free leather cross-body service dog leash. Custom made per your specs. Again, great service and excellent craftsmanship.

www.onlead.biz

Bold Leash Designs have beautiful, high-quality leather service dog cross-body leashes.

www.boldleaddesigns.com

36" training lead is made from a unique textured water resistant material. Easy grip, wipes clean, can be tossed in washing machine or dishwasher or hosed off. High quality.

www.wildrosetradingcompany.com

Zumileads offer a perfect, simple non-leather lead with color and personalization options. Well made with great support and fast service.

www.zumileads.com

Harnesses, Vests, and Capes

The Freedom No-Pull Harness has a loop on its back which gently tightens around the dog's chest to discourage pulling. The chest strap is lined with velvet, to prevent rubbing and chafing. This harness also has a ring on its front, allowing connection of a double snap lead at both points for training. Lots of color combinations. Lifetime chewing warranty.

Attach Velcro to the back of two identical patches to affix to this harness or to any leash as a nice "vest-less" option for informal outings or outings on hot or rainy days.

www.wiggleswagswhiskers.com

Ruffwear harnesses and packs are high-quality, long-lasting, professional-looking gear. The design of the Webmaster harness serves as the foundational design for all Ruffwear packs and vests. It has adjustable straps, with one leg step in design and 2 side buckles on left side. Straps maintain adjusted size in newest upgrades. The Approach pack features the same design with optional packs (for meters, low snacks, etc.), but is quite bulky.

With Palisades Pack, the pack itself can be removed. The base portion of the vest can be worn alone and is very similar in design to the Webmaster. Or, if you need the packs, they attach and detach very simply with four plastic buckles, on each corner of the base. A superb option, but, the packs are just as bulky as the Approach. If only they would design it with the option of smaller packs!

Single Track does have smaller packs, but is only available in "road construction orange," which—in my opinion—looks more like hunting garb than service dog garb. The design on this pack is slightly different, with the packs smaller and a little higher up.

You may call Ruffwear to inquire about registry in their service dog program which gives you a great discount on their vests and packs.

www.diabeticalertdog.com/store

The SitStay service dog cape is a great lightweight simple "cape-style" vest option. SitStay conveniently makes it available for purchase with patches or without. It is so simple and lightweight that the patches are easy to sew on, so I always sew my own since there are many more patch options if you purchase them separately from another location. Available in lots of different colors and even has a small zipper pocket (on most sizes), but really only large enough for something very small like an ID card. This is so small and lightweight that you can roll it up and drop it into a small handbag. I keep one in the console of my car—as a backup.

www.sitstay.com

Service Dog Tag, ID Card, and Patches

Double-Sided Services Patches have Velcro between the sides to fast attach and detach to leashes or harnesses—a quick way make any leash or harness a clear service dog accessory. A great option!

www.boldleaddesigns.com

Working Service Dog makes an ID badge with contact information. Very well made, driver's license quality. Superior service. They have some private galleries with designs available to teams from specific organizations (design includes logo and contact information for the organization). Wildrose Service Companions has quit a few design options with working Service Dog. The link can only be obtained via the organization, so that the designs with organization logos can be limited to their specific teams.

Working Service Dog also offers quite few options for displaying the ID badge. I prefer to keep mine in my wallet, but many teams chose to attach to vest with a strap or clip or ID card holder.

www.workingservicedog.com

Red Dingo offers an enamel/stainless custom dog ID Tag—great quality. Many design, color and size options. Engraving available.

www.reddingo.com

A large assortment of service dog patches are available by Clevenger Embroidery. Special orders available by contacting store. Great high-quality sew-on embroidery patches.

www.diabeticalertdog.com/store

Dog Boots
Pawz has disposable and very portable dog booties. Reusable and easy to carry.

www.petco.com

Ruffwear offersdog boots that are more bulky and less "portable," but amazingly well made and very durable. Typical Ruffwear high-quality craftsmanship. Sturdy and rugged enough for any environment. A little on the pricey side, but made to last. Slightly awkward to put on but nicely fitting and stay on well.

www.diabeticalertdog.com

Water or Food Bowl
Dexas Popware for Pets are collapsible bowls that "smoosh"

flat, accordion style. Can be attached to vest with small snap or carabiner clip or will drop down into a vest-pack or small bag. Easy to rinse and wipe clean. Dishwasher safe.

www.popwareforpets.com

Buddy Bowl no-spill dog bowls are a great option for the mischievous dog that likes to see what happens when he turns the bow.

www.amazon.com/s/ref=nb_sb_noss_1?url=search-alias%3Daps&field-keywords=Buddy%20bow

Stainless no spill bowls are easy to toss into the dishwasher after each use or at the end of the day. They don't get nicks and scratches, which can promote growth of bacteria that increase opportunity for illness for dog.

Walmart, Wildrose Trading Company

Wag.com sells portable, collapsible bowls in lots of colors and sizes and also many options on the stainless still bowl, including varieties with no skid surface or designs created to slow down the fast-eater.

www.wag.com

Note: In an emergency, your clean, unused plastic poop bag can double for a water bow. Just open and then roll the edges down to form a bowl.

Portable Crates

Firstrax Port-a-crate is well made and soft, but not recommended for chewing pups, for obvious reasons. Easy to collapse. In the event of chewing, a replacement shell can be ordered. Shell can be removed for washing and replaced without too much difficulty.

www.firstrax.net

Petsmart offers a Nature's Miracle soft crate

www.petsmart.com

Poop Bag Dispensers

Paww pick pocket pouch poop bag dispenser fits on handle of a Webmaster harness. Low profile.

www.paww.com

Alite boa pod poop bag dispenser also fits on the handle of a Webmaster harness or around leash.

www.wildrosetradingcompany.com or www.alitedesigns.com

Five star pet purse dispenser will carry poop bags or Pawz booties

www.fivestarpet.com

Miscellaneous

Kuranda Cot is an essential! It has a chew-proof, high quality design. Can be squirted clean with hose or disassembled to facilitate washing mat in the washer.

www.diabeticalertdog.com or

www.wildrosetradingcompany.com

Spibelt treat pouch is low-profile.

www.spibelt.com

Terry Ryan Treat Pouch is well made, with a strong hinge opening for ease of access and to remain open, if desired, during training sessions. Treat section as well as storage pocket. 6.5 X 8.5, water resistant, machine washable, with an adjustable webbing belt as well as belt clip.

www.clickertraining.com

Chrome bolt snaps help attach stuff to stuff.

www.jjdog.com

Bringsels come in custom ordered colors, quality material, nicely made, many color and style options.

www.diabeticalertdog.com/store

Helpful Links

www.diabeticlaertdog.com—owner, Rachel Thornton. Website mission statement: "diabeticalertdog.com will continually strive to be the best place on the net for supplies, training, advice, encouragement and honesty in the DAD industry." The site has almost a six-year history of DAD dialog.

clickertraining.com—great tabs on this site with video, how-to articles, blogs, gear, trainer info and more.

www.servicedogcentral.org—a community of service dog partners and trainers parenting combined knowledge about service dogs. Not my favorite forum, but it is a great source for legal info and state laws. The "service dog laws" sections list laws and cases by country and by state.

www.assistancedogsinternational.org—a coalition of nonprofit organizations that train and place service dogs. The purpose of ADI is to improve the training, placement, and utilization of service dogs by establishing and promoting standards within the industry.

www.dogvideoindex.blogspot.com—a well-organized collection of free 'how to' videos for training dogs using positive (force free) approaches to do basic behaviors, tricks, dog sports and service dog tasks.

There are also videos on training principles and applications, natural history of dogs, husbandry (care and play), improving your observation skills and more. Stay tuned as more video are added all the time!

www.blackdogsrule.com—Canine Hope's Frank Wisneski blogs and posts great photos from "Team Black Dogs Rule," featuring Major and Raven.

Facebook Pages
Wildrose Kennels
diabeticalertdog.com
Diabetes Alert Dogs
A Guardian Angel for Stella
Saving Luke—a Diabetic Alert Dog for Luke
Willow Wonka and Moxie Soda Pup

Where's Wuby

YouTube Channels
klsproperties (featuring Willow Wonka, Moxie Soda pup, and other dogs with which Laurie Scwhartz has assisted)
kikopup—fabulous how-to videos for many topics
Wildrose Kennels—training videos of Mike Stewart and other Wildrose Trainers
Maureen Brown—videos of obedience, public access and DAD training. All positive reinforcement only
Donna Hill—all videos organized and indexed here www.dogvideoindex.blogspot.com
A resource for service dog training.

Suggested Reading
Animals Make Us Human, Temple Grandin
Barking, Turid Rugaas
Bones Would Rain from The Sky, Suzanne Clothier
Clicking with Your Dog: Step-by-Step in Pictures, Peggy Tillman
Culture Clash, Jean Donaldson
Don't Shoot the Dog, Karen Pryor
Essential First Aid for Dog Owners, Lorrie Boldrick
Fired Up, Frantic and Freaked Out: Training the Crazy Dog from Over the Top to Under Control, Laura van Arondonk Baugh
On Talking Terms with Dogs, Turid Rugaas
Reaching the Animal Mind, Karen Pryor
Sporting Dog and Retriever Training: The Wildrose Way, Mike Stewart
The Other End of the Leash, Why We Do What We Do Around Dogs, Patricia McConnell
The Power of Positive Dog Training, Pat Miller
The Thinking Dog: Crossover to Clicker Training, Gail

Fisher

Training Levels: Steps to Success, Sue Ailsby

Training Your Diabetic Alert Dog, Sue Barnes and Rita Martinez

Working Like Dogs: The Service Dog Guide Book, Marcie Davis and Melissa Bunnell

Works Cited

The Americans with Disabilities Act. www.ada.gov.

Blakemore, Colin. *The Mind Machine.* New York: BBC Books, 1988.

Children with Diabetes. *The Dead in the Bed Syndrome.* www.childrenwithdiabetes.com/d_on_g00.htm.

Horowitz, Alexandra. *Inside of a Dog: What Dogs See, Smell, and Know.* New York: Scribner, 2009.

Pryor, Karen. www.clickertraining.com/glossary.

Rintala, Diana H; Sachs-Ericsson, Natalie; and Hart, Karen A. "Effects of Service Dogs On the Lives of Persons with Mobility Impairments: A Pre-post Study Design." SCI Psychosocial Process, 15(2): 2002 Summer: 69-72.

Sakson, Sharon. *Paws & Effect: The Healing Power of Dogs.* New York: Spiegel & Grau, 2009.

Stewart, Mike. *Sporting Dog and Retriever Training: The Wildrose Way.* New York: Universe Publishing, 2012.

Wood, Lindsay. "Clicker Bridging Stimulus Efficacy." Master's Thesis, Hunter College, 2008.

Notes on Contributors

Ben McClelland is Professor and Schillig Chair of English at the University of Mississippi, where he has taught courses in literature and writing for twenty-seven years. He has written two professional books and a nonfiction memoir, Soldier's Son. Since 2011, he has been associated with Wildrose as an apprentice trainer and blog writer. An avid hunter, his favorite sport is duck hunting with his Wildrose retrievers, Eider and Mac.

Rachel Thornton is a trainer for the Wildrose Diabetic Alert Dog (DAD) Program. Rachel's daughter was diagnosed with type 1 diabetes when she was eleven years old. In searching for DADs, Rachel and Capri were both ripped off by a scam artist before finding some Wildrose pups.

Along with Capri Smith, strong-willed Rachel pioneered the scent training methods with their dogs, Mr Darcy and Teddy Bear. They happened to be working with Wildrose dogs, so Rachel went to Mike and Cathy Stewart for help with obedience training. Voila! The DAD program was born.

Abi Thornton Atkinson, now a twentysomething wife and mom, is Rachel Thornton's daughter. With the energy and élan of a bright young woman, Abi presents her perspective on the story of her illness, growing up with Mr Darcy, and transitioning to college, work, and marriage with him. Notably, Abi used real-time training to hone Mr Darcy's scenting skills during her blood sugar level changes. Abi lives in Tuscaloosa, Alabama, with her youth-pastor husband and their four-month-old baby girl. For pastimes, Abi enjoys playing the piano, cooking, and reading.

Virginian **Capri Smith,** a married mother of four, is a secular home schooler, who likes to live by a toolbox philosophy, adding tools and skills to her repertoire as she moves through her years. A woman of awesome intellect, varied interests, and exceptional drive, Capri is a mental health counselor and a world traveler. Presently, she is writing thrillers. Lucky thing that Capri has so many positive things going for her, because she got blind-sided. Capri felt that a monster had attacked her family when type 1 diabetes ravaged her daughter, Ciara, at nine years of age. The Smiths endured many emergency interventions to save Ciara's life. The unpredictable, frantic episodes ate at the fabric of their lives. Desperate, Capri began a long, arduous journey to find help in a service alert dog. Finally, there was Teddy Bear and training help from Wildrose. Capri formed a community with Rachel Thornton and other mothers, who were learning to train DADs, to socially develop training expertise, which served as the basis for future DAD training.

Coloradoan **Devon Wright** is a senior majoring in Nonprofit Marketing at Baylor. Devon rode on the varsity equestrian team her freshman year, and still enjoys riding horses for recreation. Born and raised in Vail, she and her parents, Chris and Jen, and her two younger brothers, Mike and Andy, have always been avid outdoors people. Through her teen years, Devon sought to hide her diabetes from others. But she was very ill and unpredictably unstable. Reluctantly she accompanied her mother to a DAD workshop at Wildrose. Soon after they walked into the meeting room, a dog alerted Devon to high blood sugar. Game over. She was so impressed with these people and their dogs that she got Olive, who is trained as a gundog and a DAD. At college both she and Olive received sorority bids. Devon writes about the struggles that she and Olive have dealt with as well as the joys of going to college and of hunting with her family. Significantly, Devon learned about the subtle emotional bond between herself and Olive and how she can maintain balance in their relationship.

CSR **Megan DeHaven** lives in northern Ohio and works swing shift in a dog hospital emergency room. A bright urban professional, Megan feared death by nighttime coma and called Cathy Stewart in tears, begging for a dog that would be able to wake her when she dropped low. Enter Juniper. A keen dog handler, Megan has developed a symbiosis with Juniper that we'd all love to have with our dogs. When at work with Juniper, Megan uses hand signals to respond to Juniper's subtle alerts. Megan makes sure to give Juniper some daily recreation and Megan's favorite recreation is listening to local bands.

As a college freshman, **Sharon Stinson** knew nothing about diabetes when diagnosed with it, except that in *Steel Magnolias,* Shelby died of it. So Sharon panicked, thinking for sure she was the Julia Roberts character and headed to the grave. She also began suffering from fibromyalgia and chronic migraines that also affect her blood sugar. A lifelong resident of Oxford, Mississippi, Sharon taught special education for three years, but illness forced her to quit. Like most of these writers, Sharon experienced several late-night ambulance rides to the emergency room, until she found Wildrose Gracie, whom she and her husband trained from a pup. For five years Gracie assisted Sharon, who taught piano part-time. Sharon continued to have struggles with illness and was also challenged on access to a local grocery store by an unaware assistant manager. Sharon began speaking publicly, explaining how having a DAD literally saved and changed her life, and advocating for better education on public access laws.

Tragically, Gracie recently died in a home accident, leaving Sharon in grief and beginning life all over with a new DAD. Sharon's fate is one that all of us dog owners will face and her story presents us with useful reflections.

Texan **Angie Simonton,** a nine-year veteran kindergarten teacher, is a single mom whose daughter, Lily, was diagnosed with type 1 diabetes before she was two. Charlie, a gundog turned DAD, became her hardworking partner in helping Lily thrive. The challenges of taking Charlie to public school were at first overwhelming, but Angie persisted in working out an effective situation. With a lot of assistance from Wildrose and with adjustments in the school, this young DAD team moved to the head of the class. Lily, now six years old, loves dancing, arts and crafts, and riding her bike and scooter. An active family, the Simontons love playing at the park, taking Charlie on walks, where he also gets a few retrieves, and, of course, going shopping.

Kitty and Tim Berry and their three children are an Air Force family, living in pastoral Owings, Maryland, near Chesapeake Bay. Tim retired from Andrew's Air Force Base as a VIP Airlift Pilot. Luke is pursuing a biochemistry major at Hood College, and Matt is a cadet at the Citadel Military College. Anna Grace, the youngest, faces destabilizing challenges from diabetes and other chronic diseases. Kitty spends all of her time keeping Anna Grace healthy by attending countless doctor's appointments and hospitalizations—fifteen this past year alone. Anna Grace's service dog, Keeper, stays by her side at all times offering all of her love, dedication, and lifesaving scenting work. A key is Keeper's maturity; she is a breeding dog that was retrained for service work. Kitty tells the tale of a long journey to find a DAD that was suited to their needs, underscoring the importance of aligning s dog with the diabetic's needs.

Duane Miller, the owner and operator of a Professional Real Estate Appraisal firm in Blue Ridge, Georgia, where he lives with his wife and son. Because he covers four states

(Alabama, Georgia North Carolina and Tennessee), he is on the road regularly. As a diabetic concerned about his health, Duane sometimes fretted making another road trip. But with his DAD, Hatch, always by his side making certain that he's safe, Duane now looks forward to their next adventure together. Duane says, "Hatch is truly one of my best friends, a perfect fit for my interests in the outdoors including hunting, fishing, camping, hiking and boating."

Tom Arsenault calls New York City home. He has had varied careers, beginning with ten years in public relations for the food industry, dining in the finest restaurants with food editors, interesting them in new ideas from his clients. Next, Tom worked in hotel management, using flexible job hours to attend classes and perform as a dancer, singer, and actor. Back injuries and low wages sent him in search of his third career: floral design. He became associated with the director of floral design at the New York Botanical Garden and worked with many New York City hotels and businesses. One thing has been constant: his relationship of thirty-seven years.

Raised in Boston, Arsenault moved to New York City, where he was a long-time businessman. Following prostate cancer surgery, he developed type 1 diabetes. Erratic swings in his blood sugar sent him into a different way of life with monthly calls to 911 to revive him. He learned to know the local firefighters by name. He also became increasingly paranoid, fearful about being alone. Searching for help, he found it in the Deep South, where gracious people and, Drake, the smart dog they trained for him, brought stability to his life. Arsenault benefited especially from the work and friendship of Lisa Mayer, who served as a volunteer trainer for Drake. Among Drake's exceptional feats is giving Arsenault reliable nighttime alerts—even when it means pushing him out of bed to rouse him. Arsenault and Drake were challenged when Arsenault's cancer returned and he had to enter treatment. The medications threw off Drake's alerting for a time, but the team eventually righted itself again. Now retired and facing continuing health challenges, Arsenault is grateful for the life that Drake has afforded him.

Lisa A. Mayer, originally from St. Louis, holds a B.S. from the University of Central Missouri and a J.D. from St. Louis University School of Law. A solo practitioner in Union, Missouri, she focuses on bankruptcy (debtor practice), domestic relations, adoptions, and minor criminal matters. Her interests include gourmet cooking, training and showing dogs in conformation, obedience, agility and field trials, and volunteering as a puppy raiser and trainer for the Wildrose service dog program.

Laurie Schwartz is a retired dentist. Now residing in Colorado and partnering with her husband in life, love, home-education of three kids, a family business and pursuing a better understanding in diabetes management, the current science behind animal behavior, and service dog training. For the past four years, she has devoted much time and energy to the medical study of type 1 diabetes following the diagnosis of her youngest child, Adam. In the process of that study, she has now added the pursuit of the science behind best training practices for training life-saving skills offered by service dogs that alert to abnormal glycemic events. Laurie works daily with Adam to handle successfully their alert dog, Willow Wonka, and volunteers to help train better Diabetic Alert Service Dogs.